MAXIMISING PERFORMANCE IN HOT ENVIRONMENTS

Ensuring high levels of performance and safety in hot climates is a key consideration for sport scientists and coaches. *Maximising Performance in Hot Environments* is the first book with a project-based approach to focus solely on exercise in this common climatic condition, providing students and coaches with a clear and concise introduction to working with athletes in the heat. Rigorous in its physiological underpinnings, the book adopts a problem-based learning approach, encouraging students to engage with the science and apply it to practical, real-world scenarios.

Posing questions such as "how should athletes be monitored in high temperatures", "what are the ideal conditions for setting a world record in a 10,000 m race", and "what special considerations should be made when working with masters athletes", the book covers all key topics, including:

- The basics of human thermoregulation
- The effect of high temperatures on performance
- Heat acclimation and acclimatisation
- Cooling
- Hydration
- Preventing heat-related illness and injury

Offering pedagogical features throughout to further enhance student learning, this is a truly innovative and unique resource. It is crucial reading for any student taking classes in environmental physiology, important applied reading for any exercise physiology students, and a vital companion for any sports scientist or coach working with athletes in high temperatures.

Christopher J. Tyler is an environmental physiologist at the University of Roehampton, UK. His main research interest focuses on the role that cooling interventions may play in improving exercise performance in hot conditions.

MAXIMISING PERFORMANCE IN HOT ENVIRONMENTS

A Problem-Based Learning Approach

Christopher J. Tyler

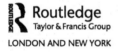

Routledge
Taylor & Francis Group

LONDON AND NEW YORK

First published 2019
by Routledge
2 Park Square, Milton Park, Abingdon, Oxon, OX14 4RN

and by Routledge
52 Vanderbilt Avenue, New York, NY 10017

Routledge is an imprint of the Taylor & Francis Group, an informa business

British Library Cataloguing-in-Publication Data
A catalogue record for this book is available from the British Library

Library of Congress Cataloging-in-Publication Data
Names: Tyler, Christopher J., author.
Title: Maximising performance in hot environments: a problem-based
learning approach / Christopher J. Tyler.
Description: New York, NY: Routledge, 2019. | Includes
bibliographical references and index.
Identifiers: LCCN 2018051618 | ISBN 9780815362715 (hbk) |
ISBN 9780815362722 (pbk) | ISBN 9781351111553 (ebk)
Subjects: LCSH: Exercise—Physiological aspects. | Heat—Physiological
effect. | Body temperature—Regulation.
Classification: LCC QP301 .T95 2019 | DDC 612.7/6—dc23
LC record available at https://lccn.loc.gov/2018051618

ISBN: 978-0-815-36271-5 (hbk)
ISBN: 978-0-815-36272-2 (pbk)
ISBN: 978-1-351-11155-3 (ebk)

Typeset in Bembo
by codeMantra

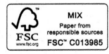
Printed in the United Kingdom
by Henry Ling Limited

CONTENTS

List of figures   *vi*
List of tables   *viii*
Acknowledgements   *ix*

1   Introduction   1

2   Basics of human thermoregulation   6

3   How hot is hot? Measuring thermal stress and strain   33

4   The effect of high ambient temperatures on exercise
    performance   64

5   The effect of high ambient temperatures on cognitive
    function   82

6   Heat acclimation and acclimatisation   102

7   Cooling   131

8   (De)hydration   159

9   Heat-related injury and illness   187

Index   *209*

FIGURES

2.1 Fictional data showing the core body temperature response to
     different exercise intensities across a range of temperatures   11
2.2 Changes in heart rate, stroke volume, cardiac output, and
     maximal oxygen uptake during prolonged steady-state cycling
     exercise in hot (35°C) and cool (22°C) conditions   13
2.3 Cardiovascular drift summarised   14
2.4 Changes in cardiac output and renal, splanchnic, and cutaneous
     blood flow with passive heating in young and older men   18
2.5 The effect that thermal perception, cardiovascular strain, and
     ratings of perceived exertion have on self-selected exercise
     intensity in a hot environment   20
3.1 Historical data of non-finishers per 1,000 starters and
     starting WBGTs   35
3.2 Historical WBGT and unsuccessful finisher data from three
     fictional races   38
3.3 Sites commonly used for measuring core, skin, and mean body
     temperature   41
3.4 Variations in resting, deep body temperature among 12
     measurement sites. Means and 95% confidence intervals for
     each total sample   42
3.5 Mean skin temperature (n = 30) during rest (four devices),
     exercise (three devices), and recovery (four devices)   46
3.6 Historical data showing the number of non-finishers per 1,000
     runners at different WBGTs   54
4.1 Mean (±95% confidence intervals) percentage change in
     performance observed in temperate (<25°C) and hot (>25°C)
     IAAF World Championship track events (1999–2011) in male
     (a) and female (b) athletes   67

4.2 The effect of increasing the thermal stress in different ways on exercise capacity in the heat 69

4.3 Nomogram showing the relationship between thermal stress (WBGT) and marathon performance decrement 71

4.4 The effects of various pharmacological manipulations in normal and high ambient temperatures on cycling performance 75

5.1 Examples of computer-based cognitive function tests 86

5.2 The human brain 92

5.3 The maximal adaptability model 93

6.1 Characteristics of physiological adaptation highlighting the accommodation reserve range and the effects of exceeding this on adaptation to heat 104

6.2 An integrated overview of heat adaptation 112

6.3 Forest plot summarising the effect [$\pm$ 95% confidence intervals] of heat adaptation on exercise performance and capacity, and on key physiological and perceptual responses 112

7.1 The percentage of athletes who reported planning to use a specific cooling strategy during the 2015 IAAF World Championships in Beijing 134

7.2 Effect sizes observed with pre- and per-cooling approaches broken down by activity (for pre-cooling) and heat stress (for per-cooling) 135

7.3 The effect size (Hedges' g $\pm$ 95% confidence intervals) of different pre-cooling approaches 135

7.4 Thermal image showing the localised cooling offered by an Arctic Heat cooling vest – note that you can see where is (darker patches), and where isn't (lighter patches), being cooled 139

7.5 An ice vest and liquid-cooled cooling jacket 140

7.6 Progressive reduction in exercise capacity observed in the heat as airspeed was reduced in the study by Otani et al. (74) 143

8.1 Estimating sweat loss and rate 182

9.1 American football player in full kit 195

9.2 Mean time taken to cool the core body temperature by 1°C 197

9.3 Representative core body temperatures during immersion at water temperatures of 2°C (a), 8°C (b), 14°C (c), and 20°C (d) for one participant (52) 199

TABLES

3.1   Weather forecast for marathon race day about here   35
3.1a Weather forecast for marathon race day   54
3.2   Worked example for calculating the physiological strain index   49
3.3   Physiological strain index classifications (50)   49
3.4   Thermal sensation scales commonly used   51
3.5   Thermal comfort scale   52
3.6   Heat stress table and recommendations for the modification or cancellation of training and non-continuous activity   58
3.7   Core body temperature assessment summary   59
6.1   Different ways to acclimate/acclimatise   126
7.1   Table summarising the most commonly used cooling strategies   133
7.1a Table summarising the most commonly used cooling strategies   152
8.1   Summary of ways to measure hydration status   163
8.1a Quick reference table – reference values, and pros and cons of the most commonly used hydration assessment techniques   164
8.2   The effect of hypohydration on physiological strain   168
8.3   Summary of point-counterpoint discussion between Hoffman and colleagues (85;86) and Armstrong et al. (87;88)   176
8.4   Quick reference – hydration strategies   181
9.1   Summary of practical cooling interventions and their effectiveness   196
9.2   Heat illness quick reference table: warning signs, symptoms, and treatment   205

ACKNOWLEDGEMENTS

This book would not be possible without the excellent work by everyone cited. Hopefully this book inspires you to embark on a career in the field of exercise physiology and that you find your own work cited in the future, or that you can use it to maximise your athletic potential to that of your athletes.

I have been fortunate to have the opportunity to work with a number of experts located around the globe – experts that have offered mentorship and collaboration. There are too many to mention but two deserve a special mention. Dr Caroline Sunderland started me on my thermal physiology journey – initially by taking me on as a university placement student (the third year of my undergraduate was a placement year), and then by supervising me for my doctorate. I would also like to mention the mentorship of Professor Stephen Cheung. An email exchange led to reciprocal laboratory visits and a number of collaborative projects – I even ended up staying at his house for a few weeks! Thank you both.

Science is an excellent career choice (Stephen once told me that a career in science was great because "you get paid to find out new things, what is better than that?" and it is very hard to disagree) but it is important to strike a balance between work and life regardless of what path you take. I am very fortunate to have been supported along the way by amazing friends and family and I am eternally grateful for their love and support. Thank you all.

1

INTRODUCTION

Maximising Performance in Hot Environments: A Problem-Based Learning Approach is a book that focuses on the effect that hot environments have on the human body, mind, and ability to perform optimally. Many people are exposed to such conditions due to factors such as event scheduling, the increased ease of travel, and the increasing global temperatures, and so the topic has wide-reaching exercise, occupational, and health applications.

Maximising Performance in Hot Environments: A Problem-Based Learning Approach is a comprehensive, up-to-date, and scientifically sound resource for advanced students, academic, and practitioners with a focus on the application of the science to the real world. The book covers the underpinning physiology associated with hot environments and the associated effects on exercise and occupational performance, and discusses the literature regarding strategies to minimise the impairments that are often observed. Due to the extreme nature of hot environments, the topic is also a great way to revise and revisit general physiological responses to exercise because the responses tend to be greater and occur earlier!

1.1 What is problem-based learning?

Problem-based learning involves solving challenging real-world, relevant problems with the help of trigger material to allow learning to be more active. *Maximising Performance in Hot Environments: A Problem-Based Learning Approach* adopts a problem-based learning approach and makes use of innovative, research-led learning and teaching strategies to facilitate active, rather than passive, learning. Each chapter contains real-world problems to give you an opportunity to apply and test your understanding. Hopefully, as you solve these problems, the information provided will have a clear context, purpose, and practical relevance.

1.2 Who is the book for?

Maximising Performance in Hot Environments: A Problem-Based Learning Approach has four main audiences: students, lecturers, athletes, and coaches.

To meet the academic needs of students and lecturers, this book provides a comprehensive, research-informed overview of the physiological responses to high ambient temperatures, how this impacts on exercise performance, whether these effects can be reversed or minimised, and the dangers posed to the athlete by heat.

Many physiology books tend to either be predominantly academic or predominantly applied, and very rarely both. Environmental physiology is a topic that lends itself to bridging this gap because high ambient temperatures are commonly experienced, the negative effects of them on performance and physiological systems are commonly observed, and there is a growing demand for scientific-based interventions in elite and sub-elite sports. *Maximising Performance in Hot Environments: A Problem-Based Learning Approach* aims to be informative and engaging, to ensure that the scientific content can easily be applied into practically relevant scenarios.

While many of the studies in the field use expensive environmental chambers, you do not need to have access to one in order to test out many of the topics covered yourself. You can easily make an athlete hot by getting them to train in the hotter parts of the day/year, asking them to wear extra clothing (waterproof trousers and jackets are especially good!), and/or heating a small room or tent – you'll be surprised by how many laboratories around the world still use these approaches! Remember that regardless of how you provide the heat stress, you need to monitor your athlete's health accurately in order to ensure that the approach is safe (Chapter 3 will help you with this).

1.3 How each chapter works

Each chapter follows the same structure to provide you with a consistent learning approach and contains the following subsections:

1.3.1 What should you know by the end of the chapter?

Each chapter opens with a short summary and bullet points highlighting what you should know by the end of the chapter. These are referred back to at the end of the chapter and tested using a self-check quiz so you can make sure that you have understood the key points of the chapter before applying the information and/or moving on to the next chapter.

1.3.2 Key terms for this chapter

A comprehensive list of thermal physiology terms can be found in the glossary of terms for thermal biology (1); however, for quick reference, key ones for each chapter will be highlighted before we get into the content.

1.3.3 Problems to be solved

At the start of each chapter, you will be presented with an example problem or two related to the content you are about to read. The problems are fictions but based on real-world scenarios. The chapter will contain the information required to solve these problems and you will be given little hints and tips on how to do so as you read. For example, in Chapter 9, you will be faced with the following scenario:

> You are the head coach of an athletics club preparing to go abroad for seven days of warm-weather training. The weather at home is cold and wet, whereas it is forecast to be warm (25–32°C) and dry where you are going. What steps can you take to ensure that you minimise the risk of any of your athletes suffering from a heat illness or injury while at the training camp? The main objective of the warm-weather training camp is to escape the poor weather back home rather than to induce any heat adaptations.

1.3.4 Quick questions

Every now and again I will pose a question for you to consider before reading on. This gives you a good opportunity to stop and think about a certain topic before finding out whether you were correct or not in the next section.

1.3.5 Content

Each chapter will make use of key historical research as well as the latest published work to give you a data-rich overview of the topic being covered. Often the literature is not as definitive as some would like you to believe – where there is a controversy or disagreement this book will give you both sides and help you to form your own informed opinion.

1.3.6 Answers to the problems posed

Comprehensive answers to the problems posed will be provided. These answers will show how I got to these answers. You may have gotten a slightly different solution, and as long as you can support your answer with relevant literature and data, then that is fine… In fact, it is great!

1.3.7 Summary

After a lot of information, it is nice to have a concise summary of the main points – don't simply skip to this bit though as you will miss a lot of very important detail!

1.3.8 Self-check quiz

As mentioned, each chapter will start with some bullet points highlighting what you should know by the end of the chapter. The self-check quiz will help you see whether these learning outcomes have been met and whether you have learnt the key topics within each chapter.

1.3.9 Practical tool kit

Whether you are in the laboratory or in the field, you should be able to make use of what you read. Each chapter will have some relevant resources for you to use in your research, consultancy, free time, or work.

1.3.10 References

All the references from each chapter are summarised at the end of each chapter for your reference. Please find the primary source cited and read the full manuscript where possible. Make use of you library subscriptions, personal subscriptions, and library services in order to find the primary source.

1.4 By the end of the book what should you know?

Maximising Performance in Hot Environments: A Problem-Based Learning Approach is an up-to-date, comprehensive resource for all things related to exercising in the heat. Each of the main chapters will cover a different topic, each with their own specific questions posed.

1.4.1 Chapter 2: the basics of thermoregulation

What happens to the human body when we are exposed to high ambient temperatures at rest and during exercise?

1.4.2 Chapter 3: how hot is hot?

Is there a difference between being hot and feeling hot? Do all people feel the heat in the same way? How do we accurately measure thermal stress and thermal strain?

1.4.3 Chapter 4: the effect of high ambient temperatures on exercise performance

To what extent does thermal stress and/or strain affect our ability to exercise? Are all exercise types affected in the same manner?

1.4.4 Chapter 5: the effect of high ambient temperatures on cognitive performance

As we get hot, or feel like we are getting hot, does our ability to perform cognitive tasks change? Are all tasks affected equally and does exercise have any role in this?

1.4.5 Chapter 6: heat acclimation

Why do many athletes undertake warm-weather training prior to competitions? What does repeated heat exposure do to the body and the ability to exercise in hot conditions?

1.4.6 Chapter 7: cooling

You may have seen many athletes using cooling interventions before, during, and after exercise – either in real life, on the television, or in the news. Why? Is there an optimal way to cool?

1.4.7 Chapter 8: (de)hydration

It seems like almost everyone carries a water bottle around with them nowadays – do they need to? What effect does hydration status have on the body and exercise performance?

1.4.8 Chapter 9: heat-related injuries and illness

What happen when an athlete gets too hot? How can you treat it and what can you do to prevent it from occurring?

Reference

1 Glossary of terms for thermal physiology. 2nd ed. Revised by The Commission for Thermal Physiology of the International Union of Physiological Sciences (IUPS Thermal Commission). *Pflugers Arch* 1987 Nov;410(4–5):567–87.

2
BASICS OF HUMAN THERMOREGULATION

What should you know by the end of the chapter?

If you have ever undertaken some exercise or physical activity in hot conditions, you will have noticed that your body responded differently than when you undertook a similar activity in cooler conditions. The reason for this is that your body was responding to the added thermal stress and strain experienced and was attempting to regulate core body temperature by dissipating the additional heat generated and stored. This chapter will cover the thermoregulatory responses made when exercising in a hot environment and will provide you with the background knowledge required for the subsequent chapters. By the time you reach the end of this chapter, you should know the following:

- How and why core body temperature increases during exercise performed in a hot environment
- The cardiovascular, sudomotor, and molecular responses to exercise performed in a hot environment
- The effects that sex, age, and clothing have on the responses observed
- The difference between autonomic and behavioural thermoregulation

Key terms for this chapter

Autonomic thermoregulation	Integrated physiological responses to heat stress made to minimise heat strain. Autonomic thermoregulation is sometimes called physiological thermoregulation.
Behavioural thermoregulation	Conscious responses to heat stress to minimise heat strain.

Clo	The thermal insulation value of clothing. The clothing required to maintain thermal comfort and a skin temperature of 33°C while at rest in an ambient temperature of 21°C is defined as 1 Clo.
Conductive heat transfer	Heat transfer that occurs between the body and a solid surface.
Convective heat transfer	The transfer of heat between you and a fluid or gas – most often water or air.
Eccrine sweat glands	The most common and widely distributed sweat gland and primarily responsible for thermoregulatory sweating.
Evaporative heat transfer	Heat lost by the evaporation of water (usually sweat) from the body.
Heat-shock proteins	Proteins that facilitate recovery from, and adaptation to, many stressors including heat.
Radiant heat transfer	The transfer of heat via electromagnetic waves.
The prescriptive zone	A range of ambient temperatures (~10–25°C) in which core body temperature will plateau during steady-state exercise.

Problem 2.1: Does age impact on an athlete's ability to thermoregulate?
You are a physiologist for the U21 national side but have been drafted in to help the Masters (70+ years of age) squad. The Masters squad are taking part in a weekend competition in temperatures of ~30°C. What age-specific considerations should you be aware of?

Problem 2.2: What should your athlete wear during preseason training?
You are the head coach of an American football team based in Texas. Preseason training starts next week and the weather is expected to be very hot (>35°C). What should you recommend that your athlete wears for contact and non-contact training sessions?

2.1 Heat storage

Core body temperature is often reported to be ~37°C in humans but in reality, core body temperature varies between individuals and fluctuates throughout the day so it is no surprise that I don't think that I have ever actually seen a resting core body temperature of 37.0°C in the laboratory! There are a number of reasons for the fluctuation in core body temperature and these are elegantly summarised in the heat balance equation (sometimes referred to as the heat flow balance equation). The equation (Equation 2.1) is derived from the First Law of Thermodynamics and describes the net rate at which an athlete generates heat and exchanges it with the environment.

The heat balance equation: $S = M \pm W - E \pm C \pm K \pm R$ (2.1)

S = storage of body heat

A positive value indicates heat gain, a negative value indicates heat loss, and 0 indicates thermal balance. It is reported in watts; however, it is often expressed relative to body surface area ($W{\cdot}m^{-2}$), body mass ($W{\cdot}kg^{-1}$), or body volume ($W{\cdot}m^{-3}$).

M = metabolic heat production

Heat production during exercise is a function of maximal aerobic power and relative exercise intensity and so differs between athletes and between sports. The heat produced is held within the body as a function of its mass, specific temperature of the tissue(s), and mean temperature and changes in the body heat content alter core body temperature. Metabolic heat production is always positive in a living organism, even at rest.

W = Work

A positive value indicates that useful mechanical power has been accomplished, whereas a negative value indicates that the mechanical power has been absorbed by the body.

E = Evaporative heat transfer

Evaporative heat transfer quantifies the amount of heat lost by the evaporation of water (usually sweat) from the body. This most obviously occurs from the skin but water is also lost through evaporation via the respiratory tract. Each litre of sweat that evaporates from the skin removes approximately 2,400 kJ of heat energy; however, evaporation, and as a result evaporative heat transfer, can be compromised by the ambient conditions if the environmental water vapour pressure is high. A humid environment has a high water vapour pressure and so in such conditions the water vapour pressure gradient between the wet skin and the environment is small. The small gradient restricts evaporation and this is one reason why it often feels hotter in somewhere like Singapore than Dubai even if the ambient temperatures are the same. Evaporative cooling is most effective when the water vapour pressure gradient is large (e.g. wet skin and a hot, dry environment); in such conditions, such cooling can account for up to 90% of heat dissipation during exercise (1) but in hot–wet environments athletes must rely more on the other, less effective, heat loss pathways. These three non-evaporative pathways (conduction, convection, and radiation) are often collectively referred to as dry heat exchange pathways.

C = Convective heat transfer

Convective heat transfer is the transfer of heat between the body and a fluid or gas – most often water or air. If you were standing outside on a cool, but not cold, day an ambient temperature of ~15°C might feel quite comfortable; however, if the wind picks up, you might feel a lot of colder despite the air temperature being the same – this is sometimes called wind chill. Now imagine that you are in flowing water at the same temperature – this will feel even colder because air is approximately 27 times less efficient at removing heat than water. Knowing this can be very useful when trying to pre-cool an athlete (see Chapter 7) or treat them for hyperthermia (see Chapter 9) as cooling will be much more efficient with water. Convective heat transfer is positive if the skin temperature is lower than the temperature of the air or water.

K = Conductive heat transfer

This is typically the net rate of heat transfer that occurs between the body and a solid surface. For example, imagine you are sitting on an open ski lift – the cold seat is at a lower temperature than you are and so you lose heat to the seat until you either get off or a thermal equilibrium is reached. Conductive heat transfer is positive if the skin temperature is lower than the surface temperature.

R = Radiant heat transfer

Radiant heat transfer is the transfer of heat via electromagnetic waves. The skin can absorb these waves from the sun directly or when they are reflected from another surface e.g. a tennis court surface. Radiative heat exchange can occur independently of air temperatures or movement so heat can be gained via radiant heat even in cold conditions e.g. on a snowy mountain on a sunny day and is positive if the environmental radiant heat is warmer than the skin temperature.

2.1.1 Regulating heat storage

There are two types of thermoregulation that work together to help regulate thermal strain – autonomic thermoregulation and behavioural thermoregulation. Autonomic thermoregulation involves a number of integrated physiological responses and, unlike behavioural thermoregulation, is an unconscious response. Thermoreceptors located in the skin (peripheral thermoreceptors) and core (central thermoreceptors) detect an increase in temperature above a threshold temperature (e.g. 37°C) and send a signal to the thermoregulatory centre (located in the preoptic area of the anterior hypothalamus) and temperature sensors located in the spinal cord. Warm-sensitive neurons are activated and heat loss pathways are initiated in a manner similar to that of a domestic thermostat; however, the mechanism whereby temperature is regulated is not quite as simple as with a domestic thermostat. A domestic thermostat uses a predetermined set point in a manner similar to the set point model of thermoregulation proposed by Hammel et al. (2). The set point model relies on the presence of a fixed central temperature from which to establish deviations; however, prolonged deviations from this set point are regularly observed (e.g. during the menstrual cycle (3)) and so Cabanac (4) suggested that the "set-point" was variable based upon the relative activity of the warm- and cold-sensitive neurons across the whole body. Mekjavic et al. (5) highlighted that a firm set point would be energetically costly (and perhaps unnecessary) because an initiation in heat loss pathways would not be required for minor, temporary increases in core body temperature. Bligh (6) proposed that the integration of this neural signals results in an overall assessment of the thermal state of the body and the initiation of heat loss or heat responses if appropriate. In this model, not only do warm-sensitive neurons initiate heat loss pathways, they also inhibit cold-sensitive neurons to prevent the initiation of heat gain/retention responses and as a result the model is called the "reciprocal inhibition" model. In the set point and reciprocal inhibition models, body temperature is the key variable and is protected within a narrow range by the switching on and off of heat dissipation/production responses. This response is easy to observe during exercise in hot environments – the exercise and hot conditions elevate body temperature and responses such as increased skin blood flow and sweat initiation are clear to see. Once exercise stops however, the extent of the skin blood flow and sweat responses reduce rapidly (7) despite core body temperature remaining elevated (and sometimes even continuing to rise). This observation does not align with the set point and reciprocal inhibition models (the heat dissipation pathways should remain active until body temperature returns to the set temperature or falls within the temperature range) and so the heat regulation model has been proposed (8). The heat regulation model suggests that overall heat storage, rather than body temperature, is the key regulated variable and so the cessation of heat loss pathways following exercise is expected due to the reduced heat production once exercise has stopped.

The body experiences greater physiological strain when exercising in the heat compared to exercising at the same intensity in temperate conditions and exercise performance is often impaired as a result (See Chapters 4 and 5 for more information on how exercise and cognitive performance are affected by thermal stress and strain). The following sections summarise how the body responds to exercising in hot conditions.

2.2. Core body temperature responses to exercise performed in a hot environment

Exercise in any climate results in heat production. This heat is produced almost immediately, and in advance of the initiation of any heat loss pathways, and so during the early stages of any exercise core body temperature starts to increase. The increase in heat storage is detected and heat loss pathways are initiated in an attempt to slow the rate at which core body temperature increases. In temperate conditions, a steady state may be reached whereby heat loss equals heat production and core temperature is elevated but stable because the increase in core body temperature is related to the metabolic rate rather than the environmental conditions. This relationship between increases in core body temperature and metabolic rate is observed in ambient temperatures of ~10–25°C – a temperature range called the prescriptive zone. During steady-state exercise, core body temperature will plateau in the prescriptive zone and only increase if exercise intensity increases (Figure 2.1). In conditions where heat generation is greater and/or environmental stress is sufficient to restrict heat dissipation, core body temperature will continue to rise.

Resting core body temperature is often stated as 37°C but even if you are resting perfectly still in a thermoneutral environment, it fluctuates throughout a 24 h period due to circadian rhythms. Typically, core body temperature is at its highest in the late afternoon/early evening (5–7pm) and lowest during sleep (4–6am) and so if you are investigating core body temperature responses of your athletes, it is important to standardise the time of measurement. It is also very important to compare core body temperature readings from the same menstrual cycle phase in female athletes, because core body temperature fluctuates during the menstrual cycle (3). Lower temperatures are observed during first ten days of the cycle (the menses and the follicular phase) when progesterone and luteinising hormone concentrations are relatively stable and oestrogen concentrations are elevated. During the luteal phase when progesterone concentrations are elevated relative to oestrogen concentrations, core body temperature increases by ~0.3–0.5°C (3;9) – peaking between the 19th and 24th day of the cycle.

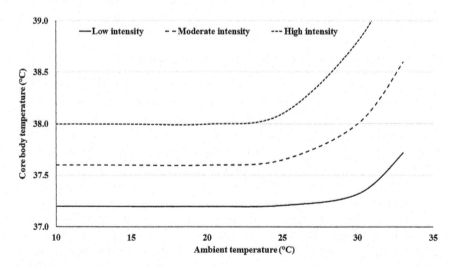

FIGURE 2.1 Fictional data showing the core body temperature response to different exercise intensities across a range of temperatures.

2.3 Cardiovascular responses to exercise performed in a hot environment

Many integrated circulatory adjustments are made when an athlete is subjected to high levels of heat stress and/or strain. The extent of these adjustments is dependent on many factors such as the intensity of the exercise, the magnitude of heat stress/strain, and the duration of the exposure.

2.3.1 Skin blood flow

When you exercise in a hot environment, you may notice that your skin becomes flushed and red in colour; this usually indicates an increase in skin blood flow i.e. an increase in the amount of blood being redirected from the core to the periphery. Once sweating has been initiated, the increase in skin blood flow serves to deliver the heat from the core which can be removed when the sweat is evaporated. Skin blood flow is regulated by two branches of the sympathetic nervous system (10). While resting in temperate ambient conditions and during dynamic exercise, the cutaneous vasculature is predominantly controlled by the noradrenergic vasoconstrictor system and endothelial nitric oxide synthase (11;12); however, when core body temperature is increased, the cholinergic active vasodilator system (regulated by neuronal nitric oxide synthase) takes over (10;11) and accounts for 80–95% of the increased skin blood flow observed during passive heat stress (13). Passive and active heating can both elevate cutaneous blood flow but passive heating does so due to active vasodilation (controlled by neuronal nitric oxide synthase) (14) whereas active heating does so due to endothelial nitric oxide synthase withdrawing vasoconstrictor tone (12).

2.3.2 Stroke volume, heart rate, and cardiac output

During exercise in a hot environment, this increase in skin blood flow means that up to 80% of cardiac output (~7 L·min^{-1}) is redistributed to the skin (15) compared to approximately 5–10% of cardiac output (~0.5 L·min^{-1}) at rest. Cardiac output can increase from ~6 L·min^{-1} at rest to >25 L·min^{-1} during exercise (16) to meet the increased demand but the large increase in peripheral blood flow means that central blood volume is reduced, compromising cardiac output and stroke volume. Fortunately, cardiac output can be protected by compensatory increases in heart rate as shown in Figure 2.2.

Reductions in stroke volume are greater when exercising in hot compared to cooler conditions (17;18) and the magnitude of stroke volume reduction seems greater during prolonged, submaximal intermittent exercise (−18% versus −10%) (18) than during shorter, steady-state exercise (−11% versus −2% (17)). By consulting the equation for cardiac output (Equation 2.2), it should be apparent that in order to maintain cardiac output when stroke volume is reduced, heart rate must be

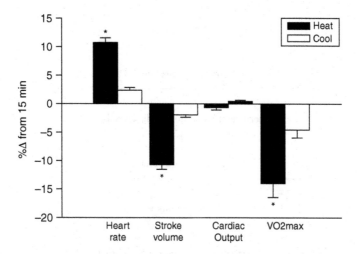

FIGURE 2.2 Changes in heart rate, stroke volume, cardiac output, and maximal oxygen uptake during prolonged steady-state cycling exercise in hot (35°C) and cool (22°C) conditions. Data are the percentage change from 15 min (mean ± SD). ★ indicates a significant difference from COOL ($P<0.05$). Figure reproduced from Lafrenz et al. (17) with permission from Wolters Kluwer Health, Inc. https://journals.lww.com/acsm-msse/pages/default.aspx.

elevated and so it is unsurprising that heart rate increases are also greater when exercising in hot (35°C) compared to cooler (25°C) conditions (17;18).

Cardiac output: Cardiac output = stroke volume × heart rate   (2.2)

During steady-state exercise in a temperate environment, heart rate responses to exercise are similar to those observed for core body temperature namely that after an initial increase a plateau is reached. During exercise in a hot environment, due to the increased peripheral blood flow and decreased stroke volume, heart rate continues to rise despite exercise intensity remaining unchanged. This increase in heart rate that is observed independent of exercise intensity is called cardiovascular drift (Figure 2.3). Unsurprisingly cardiovascular drift is greater in hot environments (17) due to the greater demands placed on the cardiovascular system and is likely to be caused by a combination of increased peripheral blood flow (19) and decreased stroke volume due to a shorter ventricular filling time (20;21). Understanding that heart rate is elevated in hot environments independently of exercise intensity is an important consideration for athletes and coaches alike because if using heart rate to prescribe and/or monitor training sessions, adjustments will need to be made when exercising in elevated temperatures. It is also important to be aware that the greater cardiovascular drift observed in hot environments reduces maximal oxygen uptake to a greater extent

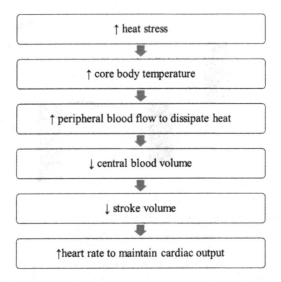

FIGURE 2.3   Cardiovascular drift summarised.

than in cooler conditions (e.g. −15% in 35°C compared to −5% in 22°C (17)) meaning that the relative intensity may be higher in a hot environment compared to a cooler one. Arteriovenous oxygen difference is largely unaffected by ambient temperatures (22–24), and so the reduced oxygen uptake appears to be due to reductions in stroke volume.

Cardiovascular drift is further increased by dehydration which places further strain on the exercising athlete because dehydration often occurs while exercising in hot environments (see Chapter 8). It has been suggested that the increase in cardiovascular drift is proportional to the magnitude of dehydration (25;26) and that the effects of dehydration and hyperthermia on cardiovascular may be additive (27), especially if dehydration exceeds 2.5% (28). Hyperthermia alone does not compromise stroke volume and can actually elevate cardiac output (29); however, exercising in a hot environment in a hypohydrated state can result in a progressive decline in cardiac output (20) despite further compensatory increases in heart rate.

2.3.3 Muscle blood flow

The increased cardiovascular strain experienced when exercising in a hot environment with and without dehydration and the redistribution of blood flow have implications for blood flow to the working muscles and to the organs. Muscle blood flow is reduced compared to control when individuals are hyperthermic ($\sim$1.0 L·min^{-1} versus $\sim$1.9 L·min^{-1}) (16) and it has been proposed that this is because the cardiovascular system does not have the capacity to maintain muscle blood flow while simultaneously redistributing blood flow to the skin (23). In order for muscle blood flow to be compromised, the strain needs to be sufficient to reduce cardiac output and mean arterial pressure (16;30). Gonzalez-Alonso et al. (30) showed that whole-body exercise, which resulted in a reduction in cardiac output of ~4 $L \cdot min^{-1}$, reduced limb blood flow by ~2 $L \cdot min^{-1}$ compared to control.

2.3.4 Cerebral blood flow

In addition to the skin and the working muscles, it is important that blood flow to the brain is maintained. Moderate exercise elevates regional and global cerebral blood flow above that observed at rest (31;32); however, it declines towards baseline levels as the intensity of the exercise exceeds the intensity required to elicit ~60% of maximal oxygen uptake or when hyperthermia is present (33;34). Unsurprisingly, dehydration further reduces cerebral blood flow (35) and although the lower final cerebral blood velocities are comparable in dehydrated and control participants following progressive exercise (~0.6 $L \cdot min^{-1}$), the lower final velocities are observed at higher intensities when participants are hydrated (~340 W) than when they are hypohydrated (~270 W) (35). Cerebral blood flow is predominantly regulated by the partial pressure of carbon dioxide in arterial blood (often abbreviated to $PaCO_2$) with decreases in the partial pressure reducing cerebral blood flow (33;36). Hyperthermia and exercise can both cause hyperventilation (an increase in breathing frequency) which lowers the partial pressure of carbon dioxide in arterial blood and it is through this mechanism that cerebral blood flow is reduced.

2.3.5 Splanchnic blood flow

Priority is given to the skin (for heat dissipation) and working muscles during exercise in the heat and so there can be a pronounced reduction in splanchnic blood flow (blood flow to the abdominal gastrointestinal organs including the stomach, liver, spleen, pancreas, small intestine, and large intestine) (29). The reduction in blood flow can increase gastrointestinal permeability and an increased movement of endotoxins such as lipopolysaccharides into the blood stream (37–39) which may result in the development of endotoxemia and/or heat stroke (see Chapter 9 for more information on heat illnesses).

2.4 Sweat responses to exercise performed in a hot environment

When body temperature increases are detected by the preoptic region of the hypothalamus, increases in skin blood flow are matched with the initiation of the sweat response – anybody who has exercised in a hot environment will have experienced this! As mentioned earlier, the evaporation of sweat is the main heat loss pathway during exercise in the heat but the sweat must be evaporated to remove heat – if the sweat remains on the skin or is removed by other means (e.g. towel drying or dripping), it does not provide any evaporative cooling. Sweat is secreted from one of three types of glands (sweat glands) located in the skin – apocrine, apoeccrine, and eccrine (40;41) – but eccrine sweat glands are the most common and widely distributed sweat gland and so are primarily responsible for thermoregulatory sweating (41). It is thought that you have 2–3 million eccrine sweat glands and that this number has been fixed since you were between 2 and 3 years of age.

Eccrine sweat glands are activated by increases in core body temperature, skin temperature, and skin blood flow (41–44) and secrete sweat on to the skin at a rate which is product of the density of sweat glands in that area and the volume of sweat secreted by each gland. During the early stages of exercise, when there is the greatest disturbance in core body temperature, much of the initial increase in sweat rate is explained by a rapid increase in the number of sweat glands recruited but once the glands are recruited the glands can further increase the sweat rate by increasing sweat secretion (45;46). The sweat released by the secretory coil of the eccrine sweat gland is almost isotonic with plasma when it is first secreted; however, the sweat secreted onto the skin is hypotonic because sodium and chloride are passively and actively reabsorbed as they pass through the sweat duct (41;47;48). The reabsorption can be impacted on by the hormone aldosterone (see Chapter 8 for more information) (49) and changes in sweat rate. Aldosterone can increase the amount of sodium and chloride reabsorbed (49) whereas faster sweat rates reduce the amount of sodium and chloride that can be reabsorbed resulting in sweat with higher concentrations of each reaching the skin (48;50).

When comparing male and females, females tend to have lower sweat rates than males if the exercise intensity is prescribed as a percentage of maximal oxygen uptake; however, there appears to be few sex differences if the intensity is prescribed based upon heat production (51) or if body size is taken into account (52). The increase in heat production observed during exercise is largely determined by the change in absolute oxygen uptake and so a female exercising at an intensity which corresponds to 60% of maximal oxygen uptake will produce less heat and require a smaller sweat response than a male exercising at the same relative workload. This holds true at intensities less than 250 W but above this females do appear to sweat less than males due to lower sweat gland secretion rates and a resultant reduction in maximal evaporative capacity (51). Notley et al. (52) showed that individuals with a lower surface area for heat exchange rely more heavily on sweat glad activation to lose heat than those with larger surface areas (who rely more heavily on cutaneous vasodilation) but that sex differences account for less than 5% of the differences in sweat and cutaneous blood flow responses during exercise in a hot environment. Amano et al. (53) reported that the reabsorption rate of sodium and chloride ions from the sweat also appears to be unaffected by sex and so it appears that males and females have a similar sudomotor response to exercise.

2.5 Molecular responses to exercise performed in a hot environment

Continued technological advancements have enabled researchers to investigate the molecular responses to exercise in a hot environment. One of the key responses appears to be the expression of heat-shock proteins. Heat-shock proteins facilitate the maintenance of cellular and protein homeostasis, and facilitate recovery from, and adaptation to, many stressors including heat (54). Heat-shock proteins can be intra- and extracellular and are classified according to their molecular weight with the heat-shock protein families weighing 70 (particularly HSP70 and HSP72) and 90 (particularly HSP90) kilodaltons receiving the most attention.

An elevation in core body temperature is a potent stimulus for an upregulation of the heat-shock protein pathways (55;56). Gibson et al. (56) concluded that in order to maximise the likelihood of inducing heat-shock protein transcription, large ($>1.7°C$), sustained (>27 min) increases in core body temperature are required and that core body temperature should be elevated above 38.5°C. Such elevations are often sought when undertaking repeated bouts of heat exposure as part of a heat acclimation regimen (see Chapter 6 for more information on heat acclimation) and so it is unsurprising that heat acclimation can elevate basal heat-shock protein concentrations (57;58). Heat-shock proteins appear to play an important role in thermotolerance (59) and individuals who have a sustained increase in heat-shock proteins following heat acclimation appear to fare better in hot environments (60;61). In an investigation conducted by Moran et al. (59), individuals who failed to upregulate their heat-shock protein expression during heat acclimation had increased physiological strain during subsequent exercise in the heat and were classified as heat intolerant (59).

2.6 Ageing and thermoregulation

In combination with the information covered previously, this section will help you answer Problem 2.1: Does age impact on an athlete's ability to thermoregulate? "You are a physiologist for the U21 national side but have been drafted in to help the Masters (70+ years of age) squad. The Masters squad are taking part in a weekend competition in temperatures of ~30°C. What age-specific considerations should you be aware of?"

The mean global ambient temperature and the global population of older individuals are both increasing. Individuals over 65 years of age have a higher rate of morbidity and mortality during heat waves (62;63) and so year on year there is an increasing number of individuals at risk during periods of sustained elevated temperatures. As discussed, the body has a number of protective responses to increases in heat stress in order to regulate core body temperature and so it stands to reason that if older individuals are at an increased risk of heat stress the effectiveness of one or more of these responses must be impaired with age.

The majority of heat-related illness and deaths observed during heat waves are cardiovascular in origin due to the great stress placed upon the cardiovascular system during such times (62). As discussed earlier, the cardiovascular response to heat stress and stress is an integrated one with many responses attempting to facilitate heat dissipation while simultaneously minimising the cardiovascular strain experienced. The increase in peripheral blood flow to facilitate the dissipation of heat is a highly effective response to increase heat stress and strain; however, in older individuals, this response is reduced (64;65) due to a reduced ability to increase cardiac output and redirect blood flow from the splanchnic region to the periphery (Figure 2.4) (64). Older individuals find it more difficult to maintain stroke volume when hyperthermic and so experience higher relative heart rates compared to younger populations in order to try and increase cardiac output exacerbating the cardiovascular strain experienced (64). In addition to having central causes, the reduction in skin blood is also caused by peripheral factors – namely a decrease in nitric oxide synthesis (as discussed earlier nitric oxide is a potent vasodilator) and an increase in nitric oxide degradation resulting in reduced nitric oxide availability (66;67).

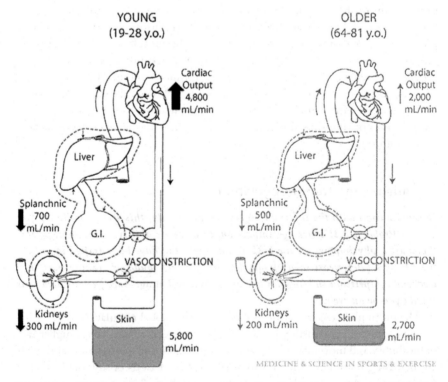

FIGURE 2.4 Changes in cardiac output and renal, splanchnic, and cutaneous blood flow with passive heating in young and older men. Figure reproduced from Kenney et al. (68) with permission from Wolters Kluwer Health, Inc. https://journals.lww.com/acsm-msse/pages/default.aspx.

Heat strain in older individuals is further increased by reduced sweat rates (69) due to a reduction in the volume secreted by each sweat gland (70) and this can elevate heat storage (71;72). For example, adults aged 60–70 years of age stored ~63% more heat than younger adults (20–30 years of age) during the course of four 15 min exercise bouts interspersed with 15 min of rest in hot conditions (35°C, 20% relative humidity) (72).

Thermal sensitivity also decreases with age (73) with a greater reduction observed in the sensation of warmth compared to the sensation of cold. The reduced sensitivity to thermal stimuli appears to start earliest in the periphery (74) and may reduce the individual's ability to behaviourally thermoregulate (see Section 2.8).

2.7 Behavioural thermoregulation

Most of the responses to exercise performed in a hot environment discussed so far in this chapter have focused on autonomic thermoregulation; however, this works in tandem with behavioural thermoregulation to minimise increases in heat storage. Behavioural thermoregulation is a term to describe the conscious responses to heat stress that are made to minimise heat strain. These responses include a down-regulation of exercise intensity, the seeking of shade, and the removal of clothing. Behavioural thermoregulation occurs in all animal species including humans and is often considered to be the first line of defence in regulating heat storage (75).

Behavioural thermoregulation is regulated by alterations in thermal comfort ("how" you feel in a hot environment, e.g. "uncomfortably hot") and sensation ("What" you feel in a hot environment, e.g. "warm") (see Chapter 3 for more information). Warm- and cold-specific thermoreceptors detect changes in tissue temperature and pass this information to the hypothalamus where the information is processed and a sense of the thermal status of the body if formed (76). Thermal sensation and comfort are both important determinants of perceived thermal strain; however, thermal comfort is perhaps the most important variable with regard to behavioural thermoregulation because while at rest thermal discomfort (the opposite of thermal comfort) is the key affective perception that provides the motivation for a change in behaviour (77;78). During exercise, it is likely that thermal comfort regulation interacts with other perceptual cues such as perceived exertion (typically measured using the ratings of perceived exertion scale) to modulate behaviour (79). While exercising in a hot environment, thermal comfort decreases as core body temperature increases (80) but it can be modified with changes in skin temperature at comparable core body temperatures such that elevations in skin temperature can exacerbate decreases in thermal comfort (81) whereas reductions in skin temperature can improve thermal comfort (77;82). Interestingly, females tend to have a greater sensitivity to changes in thermal perception than males to a given thermal stimuli at rest (83) and to warm stimuli during exercise (84) and this appears matched with a heightened behavioural thermoregulatory response (85).

Voluntary reduction in exercise intensity and/or duration is one of the most obvious behavioural thermoregulatory responses to hot environments (75;79;86) and is done (at least partially consciously) in order to reduce heat production and the rate at which core body temperature rises (87). Flouris et al. (75) proposed that the down-regulation in exercise occurs as a result of increased perceived exertion which in turn is a product of thermal comfort/discomfort and cardiovascular strain due to the link between ratings of perceived exertion and cardiovascular strain (i.e. higher cardiovascular strain results in a higher rating of perceived exertion). Figure 2.5 summarises the proposed relationships between cardiovascular strain and thermal perception (i.e. comfort/discomfort) during self-paced exercise in a hot environment. During the early stages of exercise when skin temperature, but not core body temperature, is elevated (top panel), thermal perceptions are the key modulator of self-paced exercise (bottom panel); however, as the exercise progresses and both skin and core body temperature are elevated, cardiovascular strain becomes the key driver. Thermal perceptions and cardiovascular strain interact to influence the exercise intensity selected by impacting on the ratings of perceived exertion (middle panel) (75).

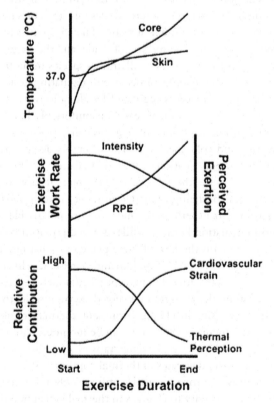

FIGURE 2.5 The effect that thermal perception, cardiovascular strain, and ratings of perceived exertion have on self-selected exercise intensity in a hot environment. Reproduced from Flouris et al. (75) with permission from John Wiley and Sons. 2015 John Wiley & Sons A/S.

2.8 Clothing and thermoregulation

This section will help with Problem 2.2: What should your athlete wear during preseason training? "You are the head coach of an American football team based in Texas. Pre-season training starts next week and the weather is expected to be very hot (>35°C). What should you recommend that your athlete wears for contact and non-contact training sessions?"

As discussed above, in many settings, an individual can utilise behavioural thermoregulation during exercising in a hot environment. The behavioural thermoregulation approach used commonly involves reducing the self-selected exercise intensity but it may also involve the removal of clothing layers. Clothing layers create a barrier between the body and the environment which limits heat loss – this is advantageous in cold conditions but in hot conditions the microclimate created can exacerbate heat strain (88). In a number of sports, clothing cannot be removed as it is required for protection (e.g. motor racing and American football) and in such situations the athlete does not have the opportunity to remove layers and so their ability to behaviourally thermoregulate is compromised.

Clothing provides insulation (insulation is a measure of thermal resistance) to the body primarily by trapping air between the skin and the clothing. As the body warms up, the heat lost to this insulative layer of air warms the air trapped here and this decreases the temperature gradient between the body and the environment reducing the potential for heat loss. Dense, thick fabrics trap more air and so are more insulative than thinner, less dense alternatives (89). The thermal insulation value of clothing is expressed in units called Clo. The clothing required to maintain thermal comfort and a skin temperature of 33°C while at rest in an ambient temperature of 21°C is defined as 1 Clo (90).

Clothing can also restrict heat loss if the clothing has low water vapour and/or air permeability. Water vapour permeability quantities the effectiveness of a material at transferring water vapour such that clothes with very low water vapour permeability (e.g. waterproof trousers) do not let water vapour escape and as a result restrict evaporative heat loss. Water vapour permeability is measured on a scale (i_m) ranging from 0 (completely impermeable) to 1 (completely permeable) (91) – an impermeable chemical protective suit has a value of 0.06 (92), whereas an American Football uniform as a value of 0.36 (93). Effective heat dissipation requires air movement and the obstruction to this posed by clothing is measured by quantifying the air permeability of the item or outfit – in layman's terms this assesses the ventilation provided by the clothing and so in a measure of convective heat loss restriction. American footballers often wear mesh-like jerseys over their protective equipment in an attempt to increase the permeability of their sporting attire – a "luxury" that some other sportsmen and sportswomen who are required to wear insulative clothing (e.g. motor racing drivers) do not have. Exercise can reduce the impact of clothing and improve evaporative heat loss by forcing air in and out of the micro-environments (94;95) and by the production of sweat. Wet fabrics have lower insulative properties (96) and sweat can decrease thermal insulation by 2–8% depending on how much sweat is retained by the fabric (97).

The majority of sport-specific clothing is composed of polyester (or a polyester mix) due to a purported superior ability to transport water vapour (i.e. "wick" sweat away from the skin) (98) and a reduced absorbance capability compared to natural fibres (e.g. wool and cotton (99). Despite the differences in properties, data suggest that there is no real difference in the thermal strain experienced when wearing garments made of natural or synthetic materials. Skin temperatures are sometimes lower, while core body temperature is unaffected (100–102). Despite having little to no effect on thermal strain, synthetic fibres may improve the comfort of the clothing by reducing the skin contact of the clothing (98) and skin irritation caused by sweat-sodden clothing rubbing against the skin (103), although the data are mixed (104–106) and this may only occur during moderate- and high-intensity exercise (101;102).

Problem 2.1 revisited: Does age impact on an athlete's ability to thermoregulate?

You are a physiologist for the U21 national side but have been drafted in to help the Masters (70+ years of age) squad. The Masters squad are taking part in a weekend competition in temperatures of ~30°C. What age-specific considerations should you be aware of?

You are used to working alongside young, healthy athletes and so it is sensible to be aware of differences between how they thermoregulate and how the Masters players thermoregulate so that you can maximise safety and performance. The Masters players are likely to be in better physical shape than your typical individual aged 70 or over, but you should still be aware of the following:

The peripheral blood flow (64;65), sweat rate (69), and sweat gland secretion (70) responses to heat stress and strain are lower in older individuals and so your players will have a reduced ability to dissipate heat compared to those in your U21 squad.

Older individuals will experience higher relative cardiovascular strain due to increased difficulty in maintaining stroke volume, and increasing cardiac output when hyperthermic (64). As a result, you may need to reduce the intensity of the training and/or incorporate this knowledge in to your tactical plans for the matches.

Older individuals have reduced nitric oxide availability (66;67) and so may benefit from increases in nitric oxide. You may wish to consider changing the players' diet or supplementing their usual diet with nitrite-rich products (e.g. beetroot) or L-arginine.

Thermal sensitivity to warm stimuli decreases with age (73) and this may reduce the individual's ability to behaviourally thermoregulate. With this in mind, you may need to do things such as prescribe shade breaks or lower intensity training sessions rather than relying on your participants seeking shade or reducing their exercise intensity instinctively.

Problem 2.2 revisited: What should your athlete wear during preseason training?

You are the head coach of an American football team based in Texas. Preseason training starts next week and the weather is expected to be very hot (>35°C). What should you recommend that your athlete wears for contact and non-contact training sessions?

Typical American football clothing (helmet, pads, trousers, socks, and shirt) has many layers and so heat loss is restricted by the many barriers created between the body and the environment. Much of this outfit is worn to offer the athlete protection and so is very important for maintaining the safety of your athlete. In training sessions that involve full-contact practice (e.g. tackle practice), the clothing must be worn, but you can still try to minimise the additional thermal load provided by the outfit. The insulative properties of the outfit can be reduced by ensuring that the fabrics used are thin (89) and that they do not unduly restrict water vapour and air flow, e.g. by wearing a mesh-like jerseys over the protective equipment rather than wearing a tight fabric with few gaps. Forcing air in and out of the micro-environments created between clothing layers can improve evaporative heat loss (94;95), and so you may want your athletes to keep moving (at a low intensity) and/or provide external convective cooling (e.g. fans) between plays. Wet fabrics have lower insulative properties than dry fabrics (96) and so you may want your athletes to dampen their garments.

During non-contact practice, you can follow the guidelines for full-contact practice but can also instruct your players to remove their helmets and padding which will dramatically reduce the insulative properties of the sporting outfit.

2.9 Summary

A complex interaction between heat loss and heat gain pathways helps to regulate heat storage and maintain resting core body temperature at approximately 37.0°C. During exercise in any climate, core body temperature increases; however, in conditions where the rate of heat generation is greater than the rate of heat removal and/or environmental stress sufficient to restrict heat dissipation, core body temperature will continue to rise. In such instances, a number of integrated autonomic and behavioural thermoregulatory responses occur to try to minimise heat gain. Peripheral skin blood flow and sweat rate increase so that heat can be removed from the body when the sweat is evaporated; however, this compromises cardiac output as a result of reductions in stroke volume and so heart rate is elevated at a given intensity (this is called cardiovascular drift). If the heat stress is severe enough, blood flow to the working muscles, brain, and splanchnic regions can be reduced compromising an athlete's performance as well as his/her health. These responses form a part of the autonomic thermoregulatory response which, where possible, is supported by behavioural thermoregulation – conscious responses to heat stress made to minimise heat strain e.g. a down-regulation of exercise intensity. Behavioural thermoregulation during exercise appears to be largely regulated by a sense of increased perceived exertion which in turn is a product of thermal comfort/discomfort and cardiovascular strain. Autonomic and behavioural thermoregulatory responses are impaired with ageing and can be exacerbated with insulative clothing. Men and women have similar autonomic responses to heat (if variables such as body mass are controlled for), but core body temperature does fluctuate throughout the menstrual cycle. Women appear to have heightened behavioural responses as a result of a greater sensitivity to changes in thermal perceptions.

2.10 Self-check quiz

At the beginning of this chapter, you were told that by this point you should have a good understanding of the following:

- How and why core body temperature increases during exercise performed in a hot environment
- The cardiovascular, sudomotor, and molecular responses to exercise performed in a hot environment
- The effects that sex, age, and clothing have on the responses observed
- The difference between autonomic and behavioural thermoregulation

In order to see whether you do now know the answers to these questions, have a go at this short self-check quiz. The answers follow the questions, but before looking at the answers, if you are stuck on any question, try looking back at the relevant section. There are a few more questions for this chapter than for the subsequent chapters, but that is because this chapter covers a lot of the foundational knowledge on which the other chapters are built.

2.10.1 Self-check quiz questions

1. Is evaporative cooling most effective when the water vapour pressure gradient between the skin and the environment is small or when it is large?
2. What form of heat transfer involves the transfer of heat between an athlete and a liquid or gas?
3. Do the physiological responses made in response to added heat stress and/or stain form a part of autonomic or behavioural thermoregulation?
4. What will happen to core body temperature during steady-state exercise in ambient temperatures that fall within the prescriptive zone?
5. During which stage of the menstrual cycle is core body temperature typically elevated by ~0.3–0.5°C?
6. Why does skin blood flow increase when core body temperature increases?

7. Why is heart rate elevated at a given intensity when exercising in the heat compared to exercising in cooler conditions?
8. Why can hyperthermia reduce cerebral blood flow?
9. What must happen to sweat for it to be effective at dissipating heat?
10. What type of sweat gland is primarily responsible for heat loss during exercise in a hot environment?
11. What proteins are expressed in response to heat stress that may improve thermal tolerance?
12. Do women and men have different sweat responses?
13. Why do older individuals have an impaired skin blood flow response to thermal stress?
14. Why do older adults typically have lower sweat rates compared to younger adults?
15. What is behavioural thermoregulation?
16. Give three examples of behavioural thermoregulation?
17. In what unit is the thermal insulative value of clothing measured in?
18. How can exercise reduce the insulative properties of clothing?

2.10.2 Self-check quiz answers

1. Large.
2. Convective.
3. Autonomic.
4. It will plateau.
5. Luteal (when progesterone concentrations are elevated relative to oestrogen concentrations).
6. To deliver heat to the skin to be removed by the evaporation of sweat.
7. Heart rate is elevated to compensate for a reduced stroke volume and protect cardiac output.
8. Hyperthermia can cause hyperventilation which lowers the partial pressure of carbon dioxide in arterial blood – the key regulator of cerebral blood flow.
9. Sweat must be evaporated from the skin. Sweat that drips off or is towelled off does not provide any evaporative cooling.
10. Eccrine.
11. Heat-shock proteins (especially those in the HSP70 and HSP90 families).
12. When comparing male and female athletes, females tend to have lower sweat rates than males; however, if the intensity is prescribed based upon heat production or if body size is taken into account, there appears to be little difference between the sexes.
13. Older individuals have an impaired ability to redistribute blood from the splanchnic region to help maintain stroke volume which compromises cardiac output. Ageing also reduces the ability to vasodilate as a result of reduced nitric oxide availability.

14. The number of sweat glands does not change with age but the sweat rates of older adults are reduced due to a reduction in the amount of sweat secreted by each gland.
15. Conscious responses to heat stress which are made to minimise heat strain.
16. Behavioural thermoregulation involves conscious responses such as reducing exercise intensity, drinking fluids, seeking external or internal cooling, removing clothing, and seeking shade.
17. Clo.
18. The movement from exercise can force air in and out of the micro-environments created between the skin and the clothing layer, increasing evaporative cooling. The insulative properties can be further reduced if the exercise is intense enough for sweat to accumulate in the garments.

References

1 Adams WC, Fox RH, Fry AJ, MacDonald IC. Thermoregulation during marathon running in cool, moderate, and hot environments. *J Appl Physiol* 1975 Jun;38(6):1030–7.
2 Hammel HT, Jackson D, Stolwijk JA, Hardy JD, Stromme SB. Temperature regulation by hypothalamic proportional control with an adjustable set point. *J Appl Physiol* 1963 Nov;18:1146–54.
3 Inoue Y, Tanaka Y, Omori K, Kuwahara T, Ogura Y, Ueda H. Sex- and menstrual cycle-related differences in sweating and cutaneous blood flow in response to passive heat exposure. *Eur J Appl Physiol* 2005 Jun;94(3):323–32.
4 Cabanac M. Adjustable set point: to honor Harold T. Hammel. *J Appl Physiol (1985)* 2006 Apr;100(4):1338–46.
5 Mekjavic IB, Eiken O. Contribution of thermal and nonthermal factors to the regulation of body temperature in humans. *J Appl Physiol (1985)* 2006 Jun;100(6):2065–72.
6 Bligh J. A theoretical consideration of the means whereby the mammalian core temperature is defended at a null zone. *J Appl Physiol (1985)* 2006 Apr;100(4):1332–7.
7 Kenny GP, Webb P, Ducharme MB, Reardon FD, Jay O. Calorimetric measurement of postexercise net heat loss and residual body heat storage. *Med Sci Sports Exerc* 2008 Sep;40(9):1629–36.
8 Webb P. The physiology of heat regulation. *Am J Physiol* 1995 Apr;268(4 Pt 2): R838–R850.
9 Stephenson LA, Kolka MA. Thermoregulation in women. *Exerc Sport Sci Rev* 1993;21:231–62.
10 Kellogg DL, Jr., Pergola PE, Piest KL, Kosiba WA, Crandall CG, Grossmann M, et al. Cutaneous active vasodilation in humans is mediated by cholinergic nerve cotransmission. *Circ Res* 1995 Dec;77(6):1222–8.
11 Kellogg DL, Jr., Liu Y, Kosiba IF, O'Donnell D. Role of nitric oxide in the vascular effects of local warming of the skin in humans. *J Appl Physiol (1985)* 1999 Apr;86(4):1185–90.
12 McNamara TC, Keen JT, Simmons GH, Alexander LM, Wong BJ. Endothelial nitric oxide synthase mediates the nitric oxide component of reflex cutaneous vasodilatation during dynamic exercise in humans. *J Physiol* 2014 Dec 1;592(Pt 23): 5317–26.

13 Johnson JM, Kellogg DL, Jr. Thermoregulatory and thermal control in the human cutaneous circulation. *Front Biosci (Schol Ed)* 2010;2:825–53.

14 Kellogg DL, Jr., Zhao JL, Wu Y. Roles of nitric oxide synthase isoforms in cutaneous vasodilation induced by local warming of the skin and whole body heat stress in humans. *J Appl Physiol (1985)* 2009 Nov;107(5):1438–44.

15 Lossius K, Eriksen M, Walloe L. Fluctuations in blood flow to acral skin in humans: connection with heart rate and blood pressure variability. *J Physiol* 1993 Jan;460:641–55.

16 Trangmar SJ, Chiesa ST, Kalsi KK, Secher NH, Gonzalez-Alonso J. Whole body hyperthermia, but not skin hyperthermia, accelerates brain and locomotor limb circulatory strain and impairs exercise capacity in humans. *Physiol Rep* 2017 Jan;5(2):e13108, doi:10.14814/phy2.13108

17 Lafrenz AJ, Wingo JE, Ganio MS, Cureton KJ. Effect of ambient temperature on cardiovascular drift and maximal oxygen uptake. *Med Sci Sports Exerc* 2008 Jun;40(6):1065–71.

18 Gliner JA, Raven PB, Horvath SM, Drinkwater BL, Sutton JC. Man's physiologic response to long-term work during thermal and pollutant stress. *J Appl Physiol* 1975 Oct;39(4):628–32.

19 Shaffrath JD, Adams WC. Effects of airflow and work load on cardiovascular drift and skin blood flow. *J Appl Physiol Respir Environ Exerc Physiol* 1984 May;56(5):1411–7.

20 Coyle EF, Gonzalez-Alonso J. Cardiovascular drift during prolonged exercise: new perspectives. *Exerc Sport Sci Rev* 2001 Apr;29(2):88–92.

21 Turkevich D, Micco A, Reeves JT. Noninvasive measurement of the decrease in left ventricular filling time during maximal exercise in normal subjects. *Am J Cardiol* 1988 Sep 15;62(9):650–2.

22 Gonzalez-Alonso J, Calbet JA. Reductions in systemic and skeletal muscle blood flow and oxygen delivery limit maximal aerobic capacity in humans. *Circulation* 2003 Feb 18;107(6):824–30.

23 Rowell LB, Marx HJ, Bruce RA, Conn RD, Kusumi F. Reductions in cardiac output, central blood volume, and stroke volume with thermal stress in normal men during exercise. *J Clin Invest* 1966 Nov;45(11):1801–16.

24 Williams CG, Bredell GA, Wyndham CH, Strydom NB, Morrison JF, Peter J, et al. Circulatory and metabolic reactions to work in heat. *J Appl Physiol* 1962 Jul;17:625–38.

25 Ganio MS, Wingo JE, Carrolll CE, Thomas MK, Cureton KJ. Fluid ingestion attenuates the decline in VO2peak associated with cardiovascular drift. *Med Sci Sports Exerc* 2006 May;38(5):901–9.

26 Montain SJ, Coyle EF. Influence of graded dehydration on hyperthermia and cardiovascular drift during exercise. *J Appl Physiol (1985)* 1992 Oct;73(4):1340–50.

27 Gonzalez-Alonso J, Mora-Rodriguez R, Below PR, Coyle EF. Dehydration markedly impairs cardiovascular function in hyperthermic endurance athletes during exercise. *J Appl Physiol (1985)* 1997 Apr;82(4):1229–36.

28 Wingo JE, Lafrenz AJ, Ganio MS, Edwards GL, Cureton KJ. Cardiovascular drift is related to reduced maximal oxygen uptake during heat stress. *Med Sci Sports Exerc* 2005 Feb;37(2):248–55.

29 Rowell LB, Brengelmann GL, Murray JA. Cardiovascular responses to sustained high skin temperature in resting man. *J Appl Physiol* 1969 Nov;27(5):673–80.

30 Gonzalez-Alonso J, Calbet JA, Nielsen B. Muscle blood flow is reduced with dehydration during prolonged exercise in humans. *J Physiol* 1998 Dec 15;513 (Pt 3):895–905.

31 Hellstrom G, Fischer-Colbrie W, Wahlgren NG, Jogestrand T. Carotid artery blood flow and middle cerebral artery blood flow velocity during physical exercise. *J Appl Physiol (1985)* 1996 Jul;81(1):413–18.

32 Ogoh S, Sato K, Fisher JP, Seifert T, Overgaard M, Secher NH. The effect of phenylephrine on arterial and venous cerebral blood flow in healthy subjects. *Clin Physiol Funct Imaging* 2011 Nov;31(6):445–51.

33 Nybo L, Nielsen B. Middle cerebral artery blood velocity is reduced with hyperthermia during prolonged exercise in humans. *J Physiol* 2001 Jul 1;534 (Pt 1):279–86.

34 Sato K, Ogoh S, Hirasawa A, Oue A, Sadamoto T. The distribution of blood flow in the carotid and vertebral arteries during dynamic exercise in humans. *J Physiol* 2011 Jun 1;589(Pt 11):2847–56.

35 Trangmar SJ, Chiesa ST, Stock CG, Kalsi KK, Secher NH, Gonzalez-Alonso J. Dehydration affects cerebral blood flow but not its metabolic rate for oxygen during maximal exercise in trained humans. *J Physiol* 2014 Jul 15;592(14):3143–60.

36 Bain AR, Morrison SA, Ainslie PN. Cerebral oxygenation and hyperthermia. *Front Physiol* 2014;5:92.

37 Costa KA, Soares AD, Wanner SP, Santos R, Fernandes SO, Martins FS, et al. L-arginine supplementation prevents increases in intestinal permeability and bacterial translocation in male Swiss mice subjected to physical exercise under environmental heat stress. *J Nutr* 2014 Feb;144(2):218–23.

38 Soares AD, Costa KA, Wanner SP, Santos RG, Fernandes SO, Martins FS, et al. Dietary glutamine prevents the loss of intestinal barrier function and attenuates the increase in core body temperature induced by acute heat exposure. *Br J Nutr* 2014 Nov 28;112(10):1601–10.

39 Zuhl M, Schneider S, Lanphere K, Conn C, Dokladny K, Moseley P. Exercise regulation of intestinal tight junction proteins. *Br J Sports Med* 2014 Jun; 48(12):980–6.

40 Sato K, Kang WH, Saga K, Sato KT. Biology of sweat glands and their disorders. I. Normal sweat gland function. *J Am Acad Dermatol* 1989 Apr;20(4):537–63.

41 Sato K. The mechanism of eccrine sweat secretion. In: Gisolfi CV, Lamb DR, Nadel ER, editors. Exercise, heat, and thermoregulation. 6th ed. Traverse City: Cooper Publishing Group; 2001. p. 85–117.

42 Nadel ER, Mitchell JW, Saltin B, Stolwijk JA. Peripheral modifications to the central drive for sweating. *J Appl Physiol* 1971 Dec;31(6):828–33.

43 Nadel ER. Control of sweating rate while exercising in the heat. *Med Sci Sports* 1979;11(1):31–5.

44 Wingo JE, Low DA, Keller DM, Brothers RM, Shibasaki M, Crandall CG. Skin blood flow and local temperature independently modify sweat rate during passive heat stress in humans. *J Appl Physiol (1985)* 2010 Nov;109(5):1301–6.

45 Kondo N, Takano S, Aoki K, Shibasaki M, Tominaga H, Inoue Y. Regional differences in the effect of exercise intensity on thermoregulatory sweating and cutaneous vasodilation. *Acta Physiol Scand* 1998 Sep;164(1):71–8.

46 Kondo N, Shibasaki M, Aoki K, Koga S, Inoue Y, Crandall CG. Function of human eccrine sweat glands during dynamic exercise and passive heat stress. *J Appl Physiol (1985)* 2001 May;90(5):1877–81.

47 Reddy MM, Quinton PM. Rapid regulation of electrolyte absorption in sweat duct. *J Membr Biol* 1994 May;140(1):57–67.

48 Sato K. The physiology, pharmacology, and biochemistry of the eccrine sweat gland. *Rev Physiol Biochem Pharmacol* 1977;79:51–131.

49 Sato K, Dobson RL. The effect of intracutaneous d-aldosterone and hydrocortisone on human eccrine sweat gland function. *J Invest Dermatol* 1970 Jun;54(6): 450–62.

50 Buono MJ, Claros R, Deboer T, Wong J. Na+ secretion rate increases proportionally more than the Na+ reabsorption rate with increases in sweat rate. *J Appl Physiol (1985)* 2008 Oct;105(4):1044–8.

51 Gagnon D, Kenny GP. Sex differences in thermoeffector responses during exercise at fixed requirements for heat loss. *J Appl Physiol (1985)* 2012 Sep 1;113(5): 746–57.

52 Notley SR, Park J, Tagami K, Ohnishi N, Taylor NAS. Variations in body morphology explain sex differences in thermoeffector function during compensable heat stress. *Exp Physiol* 2017 May 1;102(5):545–62.

53 Amano T, Hirose M, Konishi K, Gerrett N, Ueda H, Kondo N, et al. Maximum rate of sweat ions reabsorption during exercise with regional differences, sex, and exercise training. *Eur J Appl Physiol* 2017 Jul;117(7):1317–27.

54 Kuennen M, Gillum T, Dokladny K, Bedrick E, Schneider S, Moseley P. Thermotolerance and heat acclimation may share a common mechanism in humans. *Am J Physiol Regul Integr Comp Physiol* 2011 Aug;301(2):R524–R533.

55 Gibson OR, Dennis A, Parfitt T, Taylor L, Watt PW, Maxwell NS. Extracellular Hsp72 concentration relates to a minimum endogenous criteria during acute exercise-heat exposure. *Cell Stress Chaperones* 2014 May;19(3):389–400.

56 Gibson OR, Tuttle JA, Watt PW, Maxwell NS, Taylor L. Hsp72 and Hsp90alpha mRNA transcription is characterised by large, sustained changes in core temperature during heat acclimation. *Cell Stress Chaperones* 2016 Nov;21(6):1021–35.

57 Gibson OR, Mee JA, Taylor L, Tuttle JA, Watt PW, Maxwell NS. Isothermic and fixed-intensity heat acclimation methods elicit equal increases in Hsp72 mRNA. *Scand J Med Sci Sports* 2015 Jun;25 Suppl 1:259–68.

58 Gibson OR, Turner G, Tuttle JA, Taylor L, Watt PW, Maxwell NS. Heat acclimation attenuates physiological strain and the HSP72, but not HSP90alpha, mRNA response to acute normobaric hypoxia. *J Appl Physiol (1985)* 2015 Oct 15;119(8):889–99.

59 Moran DS, Eli-Berchoer L, Heled Y, Mendel L, Schocina M, Horowitz M. Heat intolerance: does gene transcription contribute? *J Appl Physiol (1985)* 2006 Apr;100(4):1370–6.

60 McClung JP, Hasday JD, He JR, Montain SJ, Cheuvront SN, Sawka MN, et al. Exercise-heat acclimation in humans alters baseline levels and ex vivo heat inducibility of HSP72 and HSP90 in peripheral blood mononuclear cells. *Am J Physiol Regul Integr Comp Physiol* 2008 Jan;294(1):R185–R191.

61 Yamada PM, Amorim FT, Moseley P, Roberts R, Schneider SM. Effect of heat acclimation on heat shock protein 72 and interleukin-10 in humans. *J Appl Physiol (1985)* 2007 Oct;103(4):1196–204.

62 Vandentorren S, Bretin P, Zeghnoun A, Mandereau-Bruno L, Croisier A, Cochet C, et al. August 2003 heat wave in France: risk factors for death of elderly people living at home. *Eur J Public Health* 2006 Dec;16(6):583–91.

63 Semenza JC, Rubin CH, Falter KH, Selanikio JD, Flanders WD, Howe HL, et al. Heat-related deaths during the July 1995 heat wave in Chicago. *N Engl J Med* 1996 Jul 11;335(2):84–90.

64 Minson CT, Wladkowski SL, Cardell AF, Pawelczyk JA, Kenney WL. Age alters the cardiovascular response to direct passive heating. *J Appl Physiol (1985)* 1998 Apr;84(4):1323–32.

65 Kenney WL, Morgan AL, Farquhar WB, Brooks EM, Pierzga JM, Derr JA. Decreased active vasodilator sensitivity in aged skin. *Am J Physiol* 1997 Apr;272 (4 Pt 2):H1609–H1614.

66 Holowatz LA, Thompson-Torgerson C, Kenney WL. Aging and the control of human skin blood flow. *Front Biosci (Landmark Ed)* 2010 Jan 1;15:718–39.

67 Holowatz LA, Kenney WL. Peripheral mechanisms of thermoregulatory control of skin blood flow in aged humans. *J Appl Physiol (1985)* 2010 Nov;109(5):1538–44.

68 Kenney WL, Craighead DH, Alexander LM. Heat waves, aging, and human cardiovascular health. *Med Sci Sports Exerc* 2014 Oct;46(10):1891–9.

69 Smith CJ, Alexander LM, Kenney WL. Nonuniform, age-related decrements in regional sweating and skin blood flow. *Am J Physiol Regul Integr Comp Physiol* 2013 Oct 15;305(8):R877–R885.

70 Anderson RK, Kenney WL. Effect of age on heat-activated sweat gland density and flow during exercise in dry heat. *J Appl Physiol (1985)* 1987 Sep;63(3):1089–94.

71 Larose J, Wright HE, Sigal RJ, Boulay P, Hardcastle S, Kenny GP. Do older females store more heat than younger females during exercise in the heat? *Med Sci Sports Exerc* 2013 Dec;45(12):2265–76.

72 Larose J, Wright HE, Stapleton J, Sigal RJ, Boulay P, Hardcastle S, et al. Whole body heat loss is reduced in older males during short bouts of intermittent exercise. *Am J Physiol Regul Integr Comp Physiol* 2013 Sep 15;305(6):R619–R629.

73 Guergova S, Dufour A. Thermal sensitivity in the elderly: a review. *Ageing Res Rev* 2011 Jan;10(1):80–92.

74 Inoue Y, Kuwahara T, Araki T. Maturation- and aging-related changes in heat loss effector function. *J Physiol Anthropol Appl Human Sci* 2004 Nov;23(6):289–94.

75 Flouris AD, Schlader ZJ. Human behavioral thermoregulation during exercise in the heat. *Scand J Med Sci Sports* 2015 Jun;25 Suppl 1:52–64.

76 Craig AD. Cooling, pain, and other feelings from the body in relation to the autonomic nervous system. *Handb Clin Neurol* 2013;117:103–9.

77 Schlader ZJ, Simmons SE, Stannard SR, Mundel T. The independent roles of temperature and thermal perception in the control of human thermoregulatory behavior. *Physiol Behav* 2011 May 3;103(2):217–24.

78 Gagge AP, Stolwijk JA, Hardy JD. Comfort and thermal sensations and associated physiological responses at various ambient temperatures. *Environ Res* 1967 Jun;1(1):1–20.

79 Schlader ZJ, Stannard SR, Mundel T. Human thermoregulatory behavior during rest and exercise – a prospective review. *Physiol Behav* 2010 Mar 3;99(3): 269–75.

80 Cabanac M. Physiological role of pleasure. *Science* 1971 Sep 17;173(4002):1103–7.

81 Schlader ZJ, Simmons SE, Stannard SR, Mundel T. Skin temperature as a thermal controller of exercise intensity. *Eur J Appl Physiol* 2011 Aug;111(8):1631–9.

82 Mundel T, Bunn SJ, Hooper PL, Jones DA. The effects of face cooling during hyperthermic exercise in man: evidence for an integrated thermal, neuroendocrine and behavioural response. *Exp Physiol* 2007 Jan;92(1):187–95.

83 Golja P, Tipton MJ, Mekjavic IB. Cutaneous thermal thresholds – the reproducibility of their measurements and the effect of gender. *J Therm Biol* 2003;28(4):341–6.

84 Gerrett N, Ouzzahra Y, Coleby S, Hobbs S, Redortier B, Voelcker T, et al. Thermal sensitivity to warmth during rest and exercise: a sex comparison. *Eur J Appl Physiol* 2014;114(7):1451–62.

85 Vargas NT, Chapman CL, Sackett JR, Johnson BD, Gathercole R, Schlader ZJ. Thermal behavior differs between males and females during exercise and recovery. *Med Sci Sports Exerc* 2018 Aug 8, doi:10.1249/MSS.0000000000001756

86 Flouris AD. Functional architecture of behavioural thermoregulation. *Eur J Appl Physiol* 2011 Jan;111(1):1–8.

87 Schlader ZJ, Raman A, Morton RH, Stannard SR, Mundel T. Exercise modality modulates body temperature regulation during exercise in uncompensable heat stress. *Eur J Appl Physiol* 2011 May;111(5):757–66.

88 McLellan TM, Daanen HA, Cheung SS. Encapsulated environment. *Compr Physiol* 2013 Jul;3(3):1363–91.

89 McCullough EA. Factors affecting the resistance to heat transfer provided by clothing. *Thermal Biology* 1993;18:405–7.

90 Gagge AP, Burton AC, Bazett HC. A practical system of units for the description of the heat exchange of man with his environment. *Science* 1941 Nov 7;94(2445):428–30.

91 Woodcock AH. Moisture transfer in textile systems, part I. *Text Res J* 1962; 32:628–33.

92 Holmer I. Protective clothing in hot environments. *Ind Health* 2006 Jul; 44(3):404–13.

93 McCullough EA, Kenney WL. Thermal insulation and evaporative resistance of football uniforms. *Med Sci Sports Exerc* 2003 May;35(5):832–7.

94 Havenith G, Holmer I, Den Hartog EA, Parsons KC. Clothing evaporative heat resistance–proposal for improved representation in standards and models. *Ann Occup Hyg* 1999 Jul;43(5):339–46.

95 Havenith G, Nilsson HO. Correction of clothing insulation for movement and wind effects, a meta-analysis. *Eur J Appl Physiol* 2004 Sep;92(6):636–40.

96 Kenney WL, Mikita DJ, Havenith G, Puhl SM, Crosby P. Simultaneous derivation of clothing-specific heat exchange coefficients. *Med Sci Sports Exerc* 1993 Feb;25(2):283–9.

97 Chen YS, Fan J, Zhang W. Clothing thermal insulation during sweating. *Text Res J* 2003;73:152–7.

98 Gonzalez RR. Biophysics of heat transfer and clothing considerations. Human performance physiology and environmental medicine at terrestrial extremes. Indianapolis: Benchmark; 1988. p. 45–95.

99 Hall JF, Jr., Polte JW. Effect of water content and compression on clothing insulation. *J Appl Physiol* 1956 Mar;8(5):539–45.

100 Gavin TP, Babington JP, Harms CA, Ardelt ME, Tanner DA, Stager JM. Clothing fabric does not affect thermoregulation during exercise in moderate heat. *Med Sci Sports Exerc* 2001 Dec;33(12):2124–30.

101 Roberts AC, Christopoulos GI, Car J, Soh C, Lu M. Psycho-biological factors associated with underground spaces: what can the new era of cognitive neuroscience offer to their study? *Tunnelling and Underground Space Technology* 2016;55:118–34.

102 Wingo J, McMurray RG. Cardiovascular and thermoregulatory responses to treadmill running while wearing shirts with different fabric composition. *Bio Sport* 2007;24:177–87.

103 Davis JK, Bishop PA. Impact of clothing on exercise in the heat. *Sports Med* 2013 Aug;43(8):695–706.

104 Brazaitis M, Kamandulis S, Skurvydas A, Daniuseviciute L. The effect of two kinds of T-shirts on physiological and psychological thermal responses during exercise and recovery. *Appl Ergon* 2010 Dec;42(1):46–51.

105 Laing RM, Sims ST, Wilson CA, Niven BE, Cruthers NM. Differences in wearer response to garments for outdoor activity. *Ergonomics* 2008 Apr;51(4):492–510.

106 Roberts BC, Waller TM, Caime MP. Thermoregulatory response to base layer garments during treadmill exercise. *Int J Sports Sci Eng* 2007;1:29–38.

3

HOW HOT IS HOT? MEASURING THERMAL STRESS AND STRAIN

What should you know by the end of the chapter?

If you have athletes about to train or compete in thermally challenging conditions, it is important to accurately measure the environmental conditions and monitor the athlete to ensure that athlete safety is not compromised and that athletic performance expectations are adjusted accordingly. By the end of this chapter, you will have been presented with information about how to measure the environmental conditions and the physiological and perceptual effect they have on your athlete or research participant. Specifically, you should know:

*   What is the difference between heat stress and heat strain?
*   How can you measure them?
*   What are the strengths and weaknesses of the various measurement options?

Key terms for this chapter

Hygrometry	The measurement of moisture in the air i.e. humidity
Humidity	The water content of the air. Humidity impacts on how hot the environment feels. At the same temperature, areas of high humidity will feel warmer than those with low humidity due to an impaired ability for heat to be lost. Humidity is measured using a hygrometer
Ambient temperature	The temperature of the air. This is most commonly reported when discussing hot environments and is usually measured using a calibrated thermometer placed in the shade.
Air velocity/flow	The velocity of the air passing over the body. Airflow impacts on convective cooling and so at the same air

temperature high wind speed will provide a greater perceived and actual cooling stimulus. Wind speed can be measured using an anemometer

Radiant heat   Radiant heat has an impact on how you feel in hot conditions and athletic settings; this is most frequently due to the sun. Exercising on a cloudy day in temperatures of 21°C can feel markedly different from running on a sunny day at 21°C.

K   Kelvin. The SI unit for temperature. 0 K is commonly referred to as absolute zero. Water freezes at 273.15 K and boils at 373.15 K.

°C   Degrees Celsius. Formally called the centigrade scales, the Celsius Scale is the most commonly used temperature scale. Water freezes at 0°C and boils at 100°C. The equation to convert temperature in degrees Celsius to degrees Fahrenheit is: °F = (°C × 1.8) + 32

°F   Degrees Fahrenheit. The Fahrenheit Scale is the official temperature scale of the United States of America and unincorporated territories. Water freezes at 32°F and boils at 212°F. The equation to convert temperature in degrees Fahrenheit to degrees Celsius is: °C = (T°F − 32)/1.8

WBGT   Wet-bulb globe temperature. Wet-bulb globe temperature combines readings from two or three thermometers to measure the combined effect of radiant heat, air temperature, and air velocity

Thermal stress   According to the glossary of terms for thermal biology, thermal stress is: "Any change in the thermal relation between a temperature regulator and its environment which, if uncompensated by temperature regulation, would result in hyper- or hypothermia" (1) i.e. environmental conditions that pose a threat to thermal homeostasis.

Thermal strain   According to the glossary of terms for thermal biology, thermal strain is: "Any deviation of body temperature induced by sustained thermal stress that cannot be fully compensated by temperature regulation" (1) i.e. a change in core body temperature caused, at least in part, by the environmental conditions.

Problem 3.1: Is it too hot for the marathon?

You are the race director and are presented with the following information about the weather forecast and previous heat illness/injury rates. Is there a risk that the event will need to be cancelled?

TABLE 3.1 Weather forecast for marathon race day

Time	9:30	10:00	10:30	11:30	12:30	13:30	14:30	15:30	16:30
	Sunny with cloud				Sunny				
Temperature (°C)	20	21	22	22	23	25	26	26	27
Relative humidity (%)	65	65	65	70	70	70	70	70	70

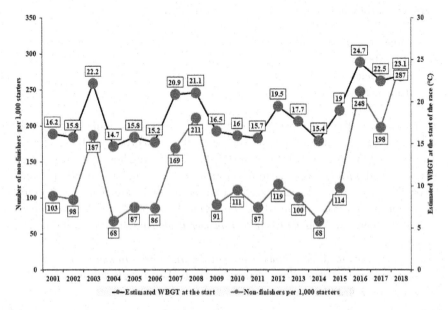

FIGURE 3.1 Historical data of non-finishers per 1,000 starters and starting WBGTs.

The marathon is scheduled to have three waves and so you will need to consider runners in all three waves:

1 Start time: 9:30am. Estimated finishing time: Less than 3 h
2 Start time: 10am. Estimated finishing time: Between 3 and 4.5 h
3 Start time: 10:30am. Estimated finishing time: Between 4.5 and 6.5 h

Problem 3.2: Preseason training is going to be hot – but how hot will your athletes get?

Preseason training is due to start and the weather forecast says that the next few weeks are going to be very hot – without access to laboratory equipment how can you monitor your athletes?

3.1 Measuring thermal stress

According to the glossary of terms for thermal biology, thermal stress is "any change in the thermal relation between a temperature regulator and its environment which, if uncompensated by temperature regulation, would result in hyper- or hypothermia" (1) i.e. environmental conditions that pose a threat to thermal homeostasis. There are a number of ways to measure heat stress but no single measure can apply to all situations (2). There are four basic environmental parameters that determine how hot the conditions feel and how much of an adverse effect they have on the human body, they are:

1. Ambient temperature
2. Humidity
3. Air velocity
4. Radiant temperature

Each of the four parameters can be measured individually but doing so offers little insight into the overall stress posed. The overall stress is a product of these four parameters and this can easily be demonstrated by comparing how you feel on a hot day with, and without, a breeze (or an electric fan) "cooling" you down. In order to try to give a more complete representation of the environmental stress, a number of approaches that combine the key individual variables have been developed.

The following sections will help you answer Problem 3.1: Is it too hot for the marathon?

"You are the race director and are presented with information about the weather forecast and previous heat illness/injury rates. Is there a risk that the event will need to be cancelled?"

3.1.1 Wet-bulb globe temperature

The most commonly used combined heat stress index is the wet-bulb globe temperature (WBGT) which was invented in the 1950s by the US Navy to set safe environmental limits to prevent the attainment of a core body temperature of 38°C. WBGT combines readings from two or three thermometers to measure the combined effect of radiant heat, air temperature, and air velocity. The three thermometers are:

1 A wet bulb (WB) – to assess the ease of evaporation. The ease of evaporation is measured by a wet-bulb thermometer, naturally ventilated, and exposed to the ambient thermal radiation.

2 A globe (GT) – to assess air temperature and radiant heat. Air temperature and radiant heat are measured at the centre of a sealed, matte-black, globe (traditionally 15 cm in diameter although many use smaller which increases the error). Globe temperature can be as much as 12–15°C higher than ambient temperature measured in the shade with a standard thermometer.

3 A dry bulb (DB) – to measure radiant heat and the effect of wind by comparing the DB temperature to the globe temperature.

WBGT is a weighted average of the wet bulb temperature and the globe temperature in conditions where the sun is not a factor (Equation 3.1) and a weighted average of all three when it is (Equation 3.2).

WBGT equation for sunny conditions:

$$WBGT = (0.7 \times WB) + (0.2 \times GT) + (0.1 \times DB) \tag{3.1}$$

WBGT equation for indoors or outdoors in un-sunny conditions:

$$WBGT = (0.7 \times WB) + (0.3 \times GT) \tag{3.2}$$

WBGT can be considered a dimensionless index (3) but is often reported as a temperature in conventional units (°C or °F). WBGTs are used as a participation cut-off for the US Army (4) and by many sporting governing bodies e.g. FIFA, IAAF, and ITF (5;6). Although WBGT is an advancement on the measurement of ambient temperature alone, there are some issues meaning that it may be inaccurate in a sporting context:

1. It does not incorporate physiological strain.
2. It does not incorporate the effects of clothing.
3. It underestimates the heat stress posed by environments that restrict evaporation (e.g. very humid conditions).
4. It responds inadequately to air movement.

Corrections apply for the intensity of physical activity, airflow, and heat acclimation status (3) but DB temperature alone might be a more appropriate way to assess heat stress in sporting settings (7). The International Organization for Standardization recommends that WBGT and the predicted heat strain model (see Section 3.2.1) should both be used. This advice is often ignored.

Measuring WBGT requires specialist equipment and issues often arise regarding the accuracy of such equipment. Portable, easier-to-use devices have become available in recent times but because they all use different algorithms and estimate WBGT based on different assumptions, the accuracy and bias of such devices vary (8). Equations exist to estimate WBGT using the four basic weather elements (air temperature, mean radiant temperature, humidity, and air velocity) in order to allow individuals without specialist equipment; however, these equations are rather complex (e.g. (9) because equations are required to model each component of the WBGT equation and so estimation tables exist to allow for quick approximation (Table 3.6).

3.1.1.1 WBGT "Do not start" considerations

Prolonged, mass-participation events such as the London Marathon attract large numbers of participants all with wide-ranging abilities – a few are aiming to break world or personal records while others are aiming to finish and raise some money for charity on the way. If the environmental conditions are forecast to be hot, there is an increased risk posed to the competitors and so the race director may need to decide whether to modify the schedule or cancel all together. The 2007 London Marathon went ahead in conditions that were warmer than usual (peak ambient temperature ~22°C) resulting in an average finishing time 17 min slower than normal. That year 5,032 runners required treatment, 73 went to hospital, and there were seven cases of exertional hyponatremia (one fatal) (see Chapter 8 for more information on hyponatremia). In 2008, when the conditions were cooler (peak ambient temperature = ~11°C), ~1,000 fewer runners required treatment (10).

Despite limitations regarding WBGT, the American College of Sports Medicine uses it to recommend "do not play" cut-offs for sporting activities. The current American College of Sports Medicine recommendation is to cancel or postpone if the WBGT exceeds 30.1°C for non-heat acclimated, "at-risk" individuals and 32.3°C for heat acclimated and otherwise healthy individuals (11). These guidelines may be too high for mass-participation events due to the large range of abilities in the field. At the Twin Cities Marathon (in Minneapolis and Saint Paul), there are only 0–1 exertional heat casualties per race when starting WBGT is < 13°C but this number reaches 11–12 per race when the starting WBGT is 22°C (10).

It is suggested that mass-participation sporting events should have the medical capacity to manage with ~120 unsuccessful starters per 1,000 runners (12% non-finishers). Based on this guide, each race should use their own historical data to establish their event-specific WBGT cut-off aiming for a cut-off of less than 120 unsuccessful starters per 1,000 runners (10). Figure 3.2

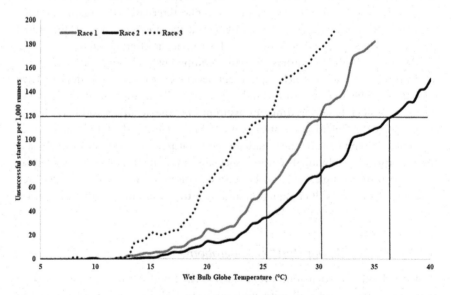

FIGURE 3.2 Historical WBGT and unsuccessful finisher data from three fictional races.

shows historical data for three fictional races, using a cut-off of 120 unsuccessful starters per 1,000 runners; it is clear that although races 1 and 2 could start with starting WBGT exceeding 25°C, race 3 should not. If race-specific historical data are lacking, non-elite races should not start when starting WBGT exceeds 20.5°C to err on the side of caution. This 20.5°C cut-off is likely to apply to any marathon near 40°N but may be lower for marathons at a higher latitude (e.g. London and Rotterdam both of which are nearer 50° N) (10).

3.2 Estimating thermal strain from thermal stress data

Direct measurement of thermal strain is essential for accurate monitoring but in many settings, physiological measurement is impractical and so a number of methods have been devised to quantify heat stress based upon predicted physiological strain.

3.2.1 The predicted heat strain model

The predicted heat strain model was developed in the 1990s and sets guidelines for heat exposure based upon predicted rectal temperature and sweat rate. As mentioned, the International Organization for Standardization recommends that the heat strain model should be used in conjunction with the WBGT in severe heat conditions (12) but the advice is often ignored. While wearing sporting clothing (e.g. short-sleeved t-shirt, shorts, socks, and sports shoes) in warm conditions (30°C, 47% relative humidity), the predicted heat strain model adequately quantifies the heat stress while walking (~165 W) (13) but the accuracy in more intense sporting situations is unknown.

3.2.2 Universal thermal climate index

The universal thermal climate index is a multi-node model of human thermoregulation, which enables the assessment of the stress placed on the body by measuring the four basic environmental parameters (air temperature, humidity, air velocity, radiant temperature) in combination with the magnitude of physical exertion and the thermal properties of the clothing worn. The universal thermal climate index appears to be better at predicting rectal temperature than the predicted heat strain model (which underestimates by 0.3–0.4°C) and is comparable at predicting sweat rate unless humidity is very high (in which case it overestimates it) (14).

As with the other measures, the universal thermal climate index was designed for occupational (15), rather than sporting, situations but it may still be useful. During the 2014 Australian Open Tennis Championship, a number of athletes suffered with the heat as ambient temperature reached ~44°C. Despite the very high ambient temperature, the conditions were under the 32.2°C

WBGT threshold to stop play (WBGT was 28.6°C). The same temperature converted to 49.6°C on the universal thermal climate index – exceeding the 46°C threshold for sporting cancellation. These data suggest that WBGT underestimates the heat stress and that perhaps the universal thermal climate index may be a better way to assess thermal stress; however, sporting data are limited.

Measuring thermal stress in and out of the laboratory: a summary

- Always use well-calibrated equipment.
- The measurement of individual environmental parameters, e.g. ambient temperature provides insufficient information to quantify environmental stress.
- Integrated models (e.g. WBGT, predicted heat strain, universal thermal climate index) give a more complete picture of the heat stress posed but sporting specific data are limited.
- The demands of the event and the experience of the participant need to be considered when assessing the threat posed by the conditions. If in doubt, err on the side of caution because the consequences can be fatal.

3.3 Measuring thermal strain

While thermal stress relates to the effect of the environmental conditions, thermal strain refers to the consequence of the stress. According to the glossary of terms for thermal biology, thermal strain is: "Any deviation of body temperature induced by sustained thermal stress that cannot be fully compensated by temperature regulation" (1) i.e. a change in core body temperature caused, at least in part, by the environmental conditions.

The following sections will help you answer Problem 3.2: Preseason training is going to be hot – but how hot will your athletes get? "Pre-season training is due to start and the weather forecast says that the next few weeks are going to be very hot – without access to laboratory equipment how can you monitor your athletes?"

3.3.1 Body temperature measurement considerations

Body temperature comprises the internal (core) and external (shell) temperatures. Core body temperature most often refers to temperatures recorded in the abdominal, thoracic, and cranial cavities, whereas the shell temperature predominately relates to the temperature of the skin.

Quick question: what do you consider to be "core body temperature" and why?

A number of methods are used to measure body temperature (Figure 3.3) – their strengths and weaknesses are summarised in Table 3.7.

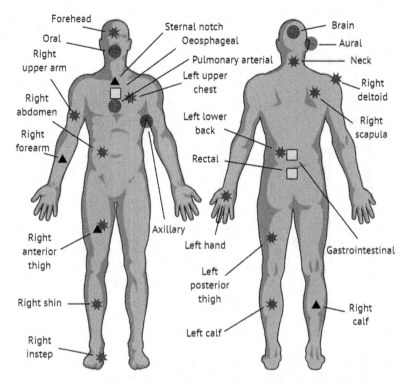

FIGURE 3.3 Sites commonly used for measuring core, skin, and mean body temperature. Circle = poor sites for the measurement of core body temperature; square = good sites for the measurement of core body temperature; star = The ISO 9886 14 sites for skin temperature (16); and triangle = Ramanathan (17).

3.3.2 Core body temperature

The ability to measure and monitor core body temperature practically and accurately is desirable in and out of the laboratory and might be critical in settings where heat illnesses may occur but what is "core body temperature"? A number of sites are measured to give an indication of "core body temperature" and each will give a different reading (Figure 3.4).

3.3.2.1 Brain temperature

Brain temperature is probably the most important core body temperature but it can only be measured in clinical settings for obvious reasons.

3.3.2.2 Pulmonary arterial temperature

The temperature of the blood within the pulmonary artery can be measured by inserting a pulmonary artery catheter. The temperature of the blood in the

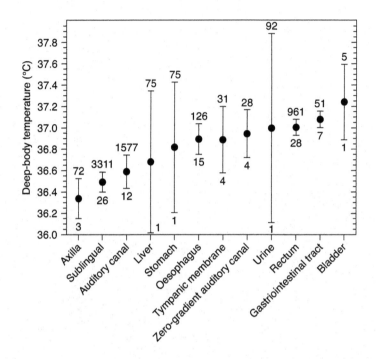

FIGURE 3.4 Variations in resting, deep body temperature among 12 measurement sites. Means and 95% confidence intervals for each total sample. Numbers above the confidence intervals are the total number of subjects, whilst those below indicate the number of contributing investigations. Reprinted from Taylor, Tipton, and Kenny (2014). Considerations for the measurement of core, skin and mean body temperatures. *Journal of Thermal Biology*. 46, 72 – 101, Copyright (2014), with permission from Elsevier.

pulmonary artery is considered the "gold standard" core body temperature due to its location; however, measuring intra-pulmonary arterial temperature is highly invasive and unsuitable for non–clinical settings.

3.3.2.3 Oesophageal temperature

Oesophageal temperature is measured using a thin, flexible temperature probe which is inserted through the oral or nasal passage until it is approximately proximal to the pulmonary artery (18). In addition to being lower than rectal temperature and gastrointestinal temperature (19), oesophageal temperature is ~0.3–0.4°C lower than the temperature of jugular venous blood (20). Oesophageal temperature is responsive to changes in temperature (21) and is often the preferred measurement site in research settings if the participants can tolerate the discomfort and difficulty of inserting the thermistor.

3.3.2.4 Rectal temperature

Rectal temperature is probably the most commonly used core body temperature in the laboratory and is measured using a thin, flexible thermistor self-inserted at least 10 cm past the anal sphincter. The pelvic area that borders the rectal thermistor is an area of high tissue density, and so more heat is required to increase the temperature; as a result, rectal temperature increases at a slower rate than oesophageal temperature and is lower than oesophageal temperature during exercise in hot conditions (21). Rectal temperature can be measured relatively easily and inexpensively but a number of barriers to the use have been reported; these include invasiveness, lack of training, lack of equipment, and lack of confidence in oral temperature (22).

Miller et al. (23) compared rectal temperature at three different depths (4, 10, and 15 cm) with oesophageal at rest, during exercise, during cold water immersion (~10°C), and during a bout of post-immersion recovery. Deeper depths were closer to oesophageal temperature and the magnitude of the difference between the two sites was influenced by the activity. The difference was greatest during the period of cold water immersion (1.72 ± 0.65°C), smaller during exercise (0.23 ± 0.53°C) than post-immersion (0.65 ± 0.35°C), and similar between all other times. It is important to ensure that the depth is at least 10 cm because while there appears to be little difference in the data recorded from thermistors inserted 10–19 cm data from thermistors inserted less than 10 cm rectal temperature is more variable (24). Temperatures measured at a depth of 4 cm while at rest can be ~0.5°C lower than those recorded at 16 cm, and although the difference is smaller during exercise, shallow rectal temperature measurements continue to be lower (24). Temperatures measured at 4 and 6 cm respond more quickly to exercise (in 0.98 and 1.58 min, respectively) than those measured at 13, 16, and 19 cm. There are few differences between temperatures at 10–19 cm, but variability is greater at 10 cm than at the other depths and so the authors recommended using 16 cm due to this depth having the highest and most stable temperatures.

3.3.2.5 Gastrointestinal temperature

Gastrointestinal temperature is a good alternative to rectal temperature during rest and exercise in the heat (25) and is measured using an ingested telemetric capsule approximately the size of a large vitamin tablet. The telemetric capsule passes through the gastrointestinal tract and transmits data to an external logger – the temperature data can either be stored or monitored in real time. Mean temperature, response time, rate of change, and peak temperature are similar between rectal and gastrointestinal temperature during rest, submaximal cycling, and recovery at 30°C; however, gastrointestinal temperature is higher than oesophageal temperature (mean difference: +0.6 ± 0.5°C) and it responds more slowly to changes (26). Following calibration, gastrointestinal temperature capsules are a valid and reliable way to measure core body temperature (27), but they can be affected by the consumption of food and/or drink, e.g. drinking cold water (5–8°C) can affect the sensor temperature for up to 8 h after sensor ingestion (28).

Due to differences between and within people regarding how long it will take to pass the capsule (differences in motility rates), it is recommended that the capsule should be swallowed at a standardised time before data collection – usually 4–8 h. Despite this recommendation, gastrointestinal temperatures are similar regardless of whether capsules are consumed 24 h or 40 min prior to running in cool conditions (~4.5°C) (29) and data from sensors ingested 3–4 h and 8–9 h before cycling and running exercise are both similar to rectal temperature during exercise (30). The ingestible capsules are generally well tolerated by individuals and do not have the discomfort associated with oesophageal or rectal temperature measurement, but they are single-use and expensive (~£50–60 each). Due to the metal content, gastrointestinal telemetric capsules should not be used in situations where the potential need for a MRI scan is high, e.g. motor racing.

3.3.2.6 Oral temperature

Quick question: when you were younger you might have had your oral temperature measured when you were ill – before reading on, can you think of any potential problems with measuring core body temperature here?

Oral temperature is cheap and easy to measure and is still one of the most commonly used ways to assess core body temperature in clinical settings. Oral temperature is often impractical for athletic settings because factors such as eating, drinking, breathing, and air temperature all affect it; however, nearly half (49.1%) of athletic trainers surveyed reported using oral temperature to measure core body temperature and they rated it as the third most valid assessment method behind rectal and gastrointestinal temperatures (22). Oral temperature is ~0.4°C lower than pulmonary arterial temperature and although expensive oral thermometers may not differ from rectal temperature during rest in the heat, cheaper alternatives give lower values (25) and during exercise, expensive and inexpensive oral thermometers both underestimate rectal temperature (25).

3.3.2.7 Aural/tympanic

Direct measurement of the tympanic membrane (a thin, cone-shaped membrane that separates the external ear from the middle ear) temperature is difficult, potentially painful, and rarely undertaken. Instead, infrared ear thermometers are regularly used, especially in clinical settings, to obtain readings. These temperatures are often incorrectly referred to as tympanic temperature but these infrared devices do not touch the membrane and so actually measure the average temperature of the aural cavity (i.e. the space within the outer ear). Aural cavity temperature can be influenced by airflow, skin temperature changes, the magnitude of hyperthermia, and the device used (25;31) and often underestimates rectal temperature at rest and during exercise in the heat (25;32). The discrepancy between sites is greatest at higher core body temperatures e.g. the mean difference was ~0.6°C when rectal temperatures were below 38°C but ~1.7°C when rectal temperatures were greater than 39°C (32) − an underestimation which could have potentially fatal consequences. William Roberts, a physician based in the United States of America, reported that when he was in charge of the "hypothermia" response team at a marathon in the mid-1990s, he called for a rectal temperature assessment on a runner who was already in the rewarming protocol because of a tympanic membrane temperature of 35.5°C. The runner had a rectal temperature of 40°C and so they promptly changed from a warming protocol to a cooling protocol (33)! Measuring aural temperature is attractive because it is quick, easy to do, inexpensive, and non-invasive; however, accuracy must supersede ease when deciding on a measurement site and so aural temperature should not be used even though some manufacturers provide a manual or automatic correction because of the underestimation.

Aural/tympanic temperature versus brain temperature
It has been suggested that because the tympanic membrane is located "close" to the stem of the internal carotid artery and to the hypothalamus (34), tympanic membrane temperature can be used as a surrogate for brain temperature. Although this practical measurement is an attractive option, strong evidence suggests that its use as a surrogate of brain temperature is incorrect (35;36). The tympanic membrane and carotid artery are separated by ~1 cm of effective insulators such as bone in an adult human and the membrane's blood supply comes from the external, not internal, carotid artery (35). Facial fanning during surgery decreases tympanic temperature; however, it has no effect on the temperature of the brain demonstrating directly the independent nature of brain and tympanic temperature (36).

3.3.2.8 Axillary temperature

Axillary temperature is measured under the armpit near to the brachial artery using a medical thermometer. It is cheap, easy to administer, and non-invasive, but provides a sheltered skin, rather than core, body temperature measurement. Axillary temperature is influenced by factors such as sweat loss, ambient temperature, humidity, and hair density and because it underestimates core body temperature during rest and exercise in the heat (25), it is a poor choice for core body temperature measurement.

3.3.3 Skin temperature measurement

The external (shell) temperature is often measured using either wired or wireless skin-contact thermistors although recent developments in infrared thermal imaging cameras have led to infrared thermometry being adopted by some

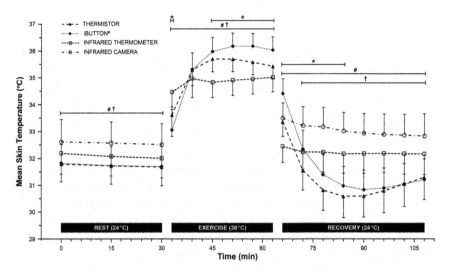

FIGURE 3.5 Mean skin temperature (n = 30) during rest (four devices), exercise (three devices), and recovery (four devices) (Data from Bach et al. (39)). Copyright: 2015 Bach et al.

laboratories. Skin-contact thermistors are typically fixed to the skin using hypoallergenic tape and/or surgical dressings, ensuring a good, direct contact to detect the conductive heat exchange between the skin and the sensor. Wired and wireless thermistors have a few practical issues such as loss of skin contact (37), the creation of a microclimate due to fixation methods (38), and the small surface area that they measure but the effect of these can be reduced with an effective set-up procedure. Wired and wireless skin-contact thermistors have acceptable levels of agreement (39;40) and because wired thermistors can be problematic due to wire entanglement (40), wireless thermistors are an attractive alternative, especially in the field.

Infrared thermometry also benefits from a wire-free set-up; however, there is poor agreement with skin-contact thermistors during rest, exercise, and recovery (39;41). Infrared devices can overestimate 39;42) and underestimate (41) skin temperature at rest compared to conductive alternatives and respond very differently to changes in skin temperature induced by exercise and recovery (39) (Figure 3.5).

3.3.3.1 Mean skin temperature

Despite being regionally variable, skin temperatures are often combined to provide a mean skin temperature. The most accurate data would be yielded from covering the entire surface area in skin thermistors but for practicality 3–15 sites are often used. The International Organization for Standardization (ISO 9886) recommends using 14 sites (16) (Equation 3.3) but due to lower intra-site variability in warm, compared to cool, conditions, 2–4 sites are sufficient for the estimation of mean skin temperature in warm and hot conditions (4–8 sites are needed in thermoneutral conditions whereas 8–12 sites are required in the cold) (43).

14-site ISO-standard 9886 (16) mean skin temperature:

Mean skin temperature

$$
\begin{aligned}
= & \left(0.07 \times \text{forehead skin temperature}\right) \\
& + (0.07 \times \text{right scapula skin temperature}) + (0.07 \times \text{left upper chest skin temperature}) \\
& + (0.07 \times \text{right upper arm skin temperature}) + (0.07 \times \text{left hand skin temperature}) \\
& + (0.07 \times \text{right anterior thigh skin temperature}) + (0.07 \times \text{left calf skin temperature}) \\
& + (0.07 \times \text{neck skin temperature}) + (0.07 \times \text{left lower back skin temperature}) \\
& + (0.07 \times \text{left posterior thigh skin temperature}) + (0.07 \times \text{right shin skin temperature}) \\
& + (0.07 \times \text{right abdomen skin temperature}) + (0.07 \times \text{right instep skin temperature}) \\
& + (0.07 \times \text{right deltoid skin temperature})
\end{aligned}
\tag{3.3}
$$

The most frequently used equation for the estimation of mean skin temperature in sport and exercise science research is probably the Ramanathan (17) equation (Equation 3.4) which uses four sites to give a mean-weighted skin temperature, favouring the upper body due to the larger surface area.

4-site Ramanathan (17) weighted mean skin temperature:

$$
\begin{aligned}
\text{Mean} - \text{weighted skin temperature} = & \left(0.3 \times \text{chest skin temperature}\right) \\
& + \left(0.3 \times \text{arm skin temperature}\right) \\
& + \left(0.2 \times \text{thigh skin temperature}\right) \\
& + \left(0.2 \times \text{lower leg skin temperature}\right)
\end{aligned}
\tag{3.4}
$$

3.3.4 Mean body temperature

The overall thermal strain experienced is a factor of core body and skin temperatures and so these data are often combined to give an estimate of mean body temperature. The equations are weighted to favour core body, over skin, temperature, with core body temperature making up 64% of the mean body temperature in the Burton (44) equation (Equation 3.5) and as much as 80% in alternatives specifically designed for hot conditions (Equation 3.6 (45)).

Burton (44) mean body temperature:

$$
\begin{aligned}
\text{Mean body temperature} = & (0.64 \times \text{core body temperature}) \\
& + (0.34 \times \text{skin temperature})
\end{aligned}
\tag{3.5}
$$

Stolwijk and Hardy (45) mean body temperature:

$$
\begin{aligned}
\text{Mean body temperature} = & (0.80 \times \text{core body temperature}) \\
& + (0.20 \times \text{skin temperature})
\end{aligned}
\tag{3.6}
$$

Take care when comparing mean body temperature data from papers using different equations – you would get very different mean body temperatures with the same core body (38.21°C) and mean skin (32.85°C) temperature depending on which equation is used. For example:

- Burton (44) mean body temperature = $(0.64 \times 38.21) + (0.34 \times 32.85) = 35.6°C$
- Stolwijk and Hardy (45) mean body temperature = $(0.80 \times 38.21) + (0.20 \times 32.85) = 37.1°C$

3.3.4.1 Changes in mean body temperature

Changes in mean body temperature are also estimated using the two-compartment model, estimating the change in mean body temperature from the change in skin and core temperatures; however, the two-compartment approach underestimates changes in body temperature during both steady-state and non-steady-state exercise (46;47). Including muscle temperature (47) or applying a correction factor (46) improves the estimation, but recording muscle temperature is invasive and even with the correction factor, only ~45–55% of change in mean body temperature is explained by changes in skin and core temperature.

3.3.5 The physiological strain index

Assessing body temperature only captures part of the overall physiological strain. In an attempt to practically address this potential shortcoming, Moran et al. (48) developed the physiological strain index incorporating heart rate and core body temperature (Equation 3.7) (Table 3.2). This strain index was a simplified version of previous models that estimated physiological strain using some or all of heart rate, core body temperature, skin temperature, and sweat rate data.

The physiological strain index uses the normalised change in core body temperature and heart rate, with each given an even weighting, to give a value between 0 and 10, which can be classified between "no strain" and "very high strain" (Table 3.3).

Physiological strain index (48):

$$\text{Physiological Strain Index} = 5 \times ((\text{core body temperature}_t - \text{core body temperature}_0) / (39.5 - \text{core body temperature}_0))$$
$$+ 5 \times ((\text{heart rate}_t - \text{heart rate}_0) / (180 - \text{heart rate}_0))$$

$$(3.7)$$

In the above equation, 0 are measurements taken at the start of the exposure and t are the measurements taken at any equal time after that. For example:

The physiological strain index was designed with maximum limits for core body temperature (39.5°C) and heart rate (180 b·min^{-1}) on the assumption that these maximums are universal; however, well-trained athletes can achieve values in excess of these. If using the physiological strain index with athletes achieving core body temperatures and/or heart rates in excess of these values, the predefined "maximum" values should be replaced with actual maximal values if possible (49). For example

TABLE 3.2 Worked example for calculating the physiological strain index

	0 min	*25 min*
Rectal temperature (°C)	36.87	38.21
Heart rate (b·min⁻¹)	62	135
Physiological strain index at 25 min =	$(5 \times ((38.21 - 36.87)/(39.5 - 36.87))) + (5 \times ((135 - 62)/(180 - 62)))$ $(5 \times (1.34/2.63)) + (5 \times (73/118))$ $(5 \times 0.51) + (5 \times 62)$ $2.55 + 3.09$ 5.64 (or 5.6)	

Physiological strain index (48):

$$\text{Physiological Strain Index} = 5 \times ((\text{core body temperature}_t - \text{core body temperature}_0)/(39.97 - \text{core body temperature}_0))$$
$$+ 5 \times ((\text{heart rate}_t - \text{heart rate}_0)/(193 - \text{heart rate}_0))$$

(3.7a)

Recommendations for measuring thermal strain:

- Always use well-calibrated, thermistors and apply correction factors when required.
- For core body temperature, use oesophageal temperature where possible. Rectal and gastrointestinal temperatures are suitable alternatives.
- Do not use oral, aural, tympanic, or axillary temperature for core body temperature assessment.
- Do not use gastrointestinal temperature if there is a high risk of an MRI scan being required before the capsule has been passed.
- Ensure gastrointestinal temperature capsules are ingested at the same time before each trial for each participant.

TABLE 3.3 Physiological strain index classifications (50)

Strain level	*Physiological strain index*
	0
No/little	1
	2
Low	3
	4
Moderate	5
	6
High	7
	8
Very high	9
	10

- Use wired or wireless skin–contact conductive thermistors for skin temperature assessment.
- Ensure that skin thermistor placement is consistent due to regional variation in skin temperature.
- Ensure that skin thermistors remain in good close contact with the skin but use as little fixation as possible. You will need to strike a balance between maintaining a good contact and not over-fixing, especially for sweaty athletes.
- While calculating mean skin temperature, or comparing your mean data with that of others, make sure that the same equation is used.

3.4 Measuring perceived thermal strain and comfort

In addition to objectively measuring thermal strain, it is important to consider how the athlete perceives these data; for example, does it matter if the athlete is physiologically hot if he/she feels cool or vice versa?

How the athlete feels during exercise in the heat can be categorised by measuring two different, constructs – thermal sensation and thermal comfort.

Quick question: Before reading on, what do you think the difference is between thermal comfort and thermal sensation?

3.4.1 Thermal sensation

Thermal sensation quantifies the perception of temperature i.e. "what" (e.g. warm) not "how" (e.g. uncomfortable) an athlete feels. The perception of temperature results from the stimulation of peripheral and central thermoreceptors, although thermal sensation is predominantly altered due to the stimulation of peripheral thermoreceptors by changes in ambient air and skin temperatures (50). For example, Schlader et al. (51) reported that thermal sensation was reduced when skin temperature was decreased, despite continued increases in core body temperature. Interestingly, thermal sensation is blunted during exercise, and greater changes in skin temperature are required to change thermal sensation by a similar magnitude during exercise than at rest; this blunting is more pronounced in men than women (52).

A number of scales have been used to measure thermal sensation (Table 3.4). In one of the earliest, Gagge et al. (53) used a seven-point scale ranging from 1 (Cold) to 7 (Hot); however, this mixed thermal sensation with thermal comfort and so in later scales "comfortable" was replaced with "neutral" (50;54;55). A more recent scale devised by the US Military reverted back to "comfortable" (56).

3.4.2 Thermal comfort

In contrast to thermal sensation, thermal comfort is "how" (e.g. uncomfortable) not "what" (e.g. warm) an athlete feels. The American Society of Heating, Refrigerating and Air-Conditioning Engineers (ASHRAE) Standard 55 (55)

TABLE 3.4 Thermal sensation scales commonly used

	Gagge et al. (54)	Gagge et al. (51)	ASHRAE (55, 56)	Extended ASHRAE	Young et al. (57)
Unbearably Cold					0
Very cold				−4	1
Cold	1	1	−3	−3	2
Cool	2	2	−2	−2	3
Slightly cool	3	3	−1	−1	–
Comfortable	4	–	–	–	4
Neutral	–	4	0	0	–
Slightly warm	5	5	1	1	
Warm	6	6	2	2	5
Hot	7	7	3	3	6
Very hot				4	7
Unbearably hot					8

defines thermal comfort as "that condition of mind that expresses satisfaction with the thermal environment" and it is thought that thermal comfort, or discomfort, is likely to be the main driver behind behavioural thermoregulation (57). Thermal comfort has been a key variable investigated in occupational settings (e.g. trying to find the ideal conditions for factory workers to maximise production) but most of the literature has focused on what conditions produce it rather than why it is perceived. As a result, our understanding on why thermal comfort (or discomfort) is perceived is limited, but it also appears to be strongly linked to skin and core body temperature. Thermal comfort appears to be achieved when a heat stimulus minimises body heat storage (58), and in normothermic conditions, skin temperature appears to be the main determinant with core body temperature playing little role (53). During exercise in the heat, core temperature becomes a key driver, and increases in core body temperature decrease thermal comfort unless skin temperature reductions also occur (51;59). During exercise, changes in thermal comfort are also related to changes in skin blood flow and sweating response (50) with skin wetness being perceived via thermal- and mechano-afferent signals as uncomfortable (60). Fewer scales exist to assess thermal comfort, the most commonly used is the scale composed by Gagge et al. (53) (Table 3.5).

TABLE 3.5 Thermal comfort scale

Gagge et al. (53)	
4	Very uncomfortable
3	Uncomfortable
2	Slightly uncomfortable
1	Comfortable

3.4.3 Perception-based heat strain index

In an attempt to address the limitations of the physiological strain index characterised by the lack of any data regarding perceived thermal strain, Tikuisis et al. (49) devised the perception-based heat strain index (Equation 3.8).

Perception-based heat strain index (49):

$$\text{Perception} - \text{based Heat Strain Index} = (5 \times (\text{TS}_t - 7) / 6) + \left(5 \times \left(\text{PE}_t / 10\right)\right)$$

(3.8)

In the above equation, TS represents a modified version of the Gagge et al. (53), thermal sensation scale is in the range from 7 "comfortable" to 13 "intolerably hot", while PE is a modified version of the Borg (61) rating of physical exertion on a scale of 0–10. When compared to the physiological strain index, the perception-based heat strain index reveals that well-trained athletes underestimate the physiological strain, whereas for untrained individuals, the perceived thermal strain closely matches the physiological strain (49). While the idea of modelling perceived thermal strain is a good one, the models to date are not perfect, for example; hopefully you have noticed that the modified version of Gagge et al. (53) scale mixes thermal comfort and thermal sensation!

Recommendations for measuring perceived thermal strain and comfort:

- Use thermal comfort and thermal sensation scales to capture "what" and "how" the athlete feels.
- Take care to familiarise your athlete/participant with the scales prior to use.
- Use the same scales to allow for comparison between experiments/training sessions.
- Take care when comparing published data – which scale did they use?
- Regional variations in thermal sensitivity should be considered when collecting data, especially when the intervention specifically targets an area of the body e.g. if you ask the athlete to rate the cooling offered by a cooling vest, are you interested in whole-body thermal sensation or the thermal sensation of the torso, or both?

Problem 3.1 revisited: Is it too hot for the marathon?

You are the race director and are presented with the following information about the weather fore-cast and previous heat illness/injury rates. Is there a risk that the event will need to be cancelled?

The marathon is scheduled to have three waves and so you will need to consider runners in all three waves:

1 *Start time: 9:30am. Estimated finishing time: Less than 3 h*
2 *Start time: 10am. Estimated finishing time: Between 3 and 4.5 h*
3 *Start time: 10:30am. Estimated finishing time: Between 4.5 and 6.5 h*

What should you do with the information provided? Although not ideal, WBGT is routinely used to establish cut-off temperatures for cancellation, so it would be a good idea to convert the data that you have to WBGT. You are missing some of the crucial data, so will need to estimate it using Table 3.1a. The estimated WBGT for each time is plotted below with the estimated time on the course for the three waves:

TABLE 3.1 Weather forecast for marathon race day

Time	9:30	10:00	10:30	11:30	12:30	13:30	14:30	15:30	16:30
	Sunny with cloud					Sunny			
Temperature (°C)	20	21	22	22	23	25	26	26	27
Relative humidity (%)	65	65	65	70	70	70	70	70	70

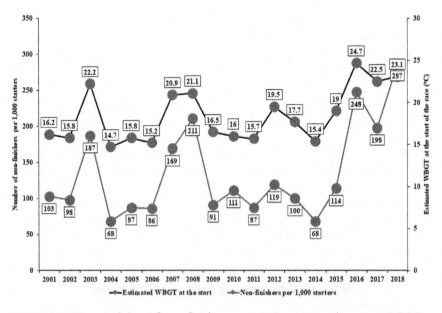

FIGURE 3.1 Historical data of non-finishers per 1,000 starters and starting WBGTs.

TABLE 3.1A Weather forecast for marathon race day

Time	9:30	10:00	10:30	11:30	12:30	13:30	14:30	15:30	16:30
	Sunny with cloud				Sunny				
Temperature (°C)	20	21	22	22	23	25	26	26	27
Relative humidity (%)	65	65	65	70	70	70	70	70	70
Estimated WBGT (°C)	21	22	23	24	25	27	28	28	29

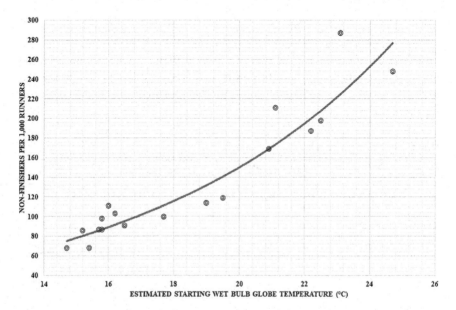

FIGURE 3.6 Historical data showing the number of non-finishers per 1,000 runners at different WBGTs.

The estimated WBGTs do not exceed the suggested cut-offs of 30.1°C for unacclimated, at-risk individuals (wave 3) and 32.3°C for heat acclimated and otherwise healthy individuals (13) (Wave 1) at any time but they do exceed the 20.5°C "do not start" threshold proposed elsewhere (10). Fortunately, the marathon has been running for a number of years and so you have the historical data regarding non-finishers and starting WBGT (Figure 3.6).

Using these data (redrawn from data already seen in Figure 3.1), the recommendation should be that the race should be cancelled or rescheduled because it is likely that the recommended 120 non-finishers per 1,000 starters threshold would be exceeded with starting WBGTs in excess of ~18.5°C and the predicted starting WBGTs are 21–23°C. Wave 3 will be the highest risk category as they will be facing the highest temperatures – one option to consider would be to move the starting time forward by a few hours if the starting WBGTs earlier would fall below the race-specific 18.5°C threshold.

Problem 3.2 revisited: Preseason training is going to be hot – but how hot will your athletes get?

Preseason training is due to start and the weather forecast says that the next few weeks are going to be very hot – without access to laboratory equipment, how can you monitor your athletes?

The only currently available practical way of measuring core body temperature directly is gastrointestinal temperature and so if the budget allows, this is a good option for direct measurement. The cheaper, practical devices (e.g. oral and aural thermometers) are not accurate enough to provide you with a meaningful and valid measurement and so should be avoided. If the budget does not stretch to ingestible capsules for gastrointestinal temperature assessment (or if the sport is too dangerous to justify its use e.g. motor racing and the potential MRI scan requirement), you should make use of the perceptual scales available. Make every effort to ensure that the athlete provides you with accurate values and does not feel pressured into providing values that under-report the actual perceived level of thermal strain.

3.5 Summary

Thermal homeostasis during exercise in hot conditions can be compromised by external and internal factors. Internally, endogenous heat production during exercise elevates core body temperature and this increase is referred to as thermal strain. The level of thermal strain can be exacerbated by environmental factors such as ambient temperature, humidity, airflow, and radiation from the sun and non-environmental factors such as clothing. Collectively, these factors provide a thermal stress. The factors associated with thermal stress can be measured individually, but the overall stress is dependent on how the factors interact (e.g. 30°C ambient temperature on a day with no wind provides a higher thermal stress than 30°C ambient temperature with an air-flow of 4 m s^{-1}) and so integrated models, such as WBGTs, predicted heat strain, and universal thermal climate index are preferred.

In addition to monitoring the thermal stress, it is important to be able to accurately measure the thermal strain experienced because high core body temperatures can compromise exercise performance and athlete health. Core body temperature measurements can be made at a number of different sites and with a range of products and the temperature readings made will differ between sites and products. Brain temperature and the temperature of the blood within the pulmonary arterial temperature are considered the most important temperatures; however, the measurement of such temperatures can only be achieved in clinical settings. Of the sites available to researchers and practitioners, oesophageal, rectal, and gastrointestinal temperatures are recommended. These temperatures can be supplemented with assessment of mean-weighted skin temperature to give a more complete picture of the extent of thermal strain experienced.

Finally, in addition to actual thermal strain, it is useful to measure perceived thermal strain. Exercise regulation is controlled to some degree by how and what the athlete feels and so quantifying this is of use – especially when interventions only change perceived, rather than actual, thermal strain (e.g. menthol application – see Chapter 7). Thermal sensation ("what" an individual feels when exercising or resting in a hot environment) and thermal comfort ("how" an individual feels when exercising or resting in a hot environment) can be measured using validated scales either in isolation or alongside physiological assessment.

3.6 Self-check quiz

At the beginning of this chapter, you were told that by this point you should know the answers to the following broad questions:

- What is the difference between heat stress and heat strain?
- How can you measure them?
- What are the pros and cons of the various measurement options?

In order to see whether you do now know the answers to these questions, have a go at this short self-check quiz. The answers follow the questions, but before looking at the answers, if you are stuck on any question, try looking back at the relevant section. For help with questions 1–4 take another look at Sections 3.1 and 3.2, if you are stuck on questions 5–8 take another look at Section 3.3, and if questions 8–10 are causing you a headache the answers can be found in Section 3.4.

3.6.1 Self-check quiz questions

1. What is the difference between thermal stress and thermal strain?
2. What are the four basic environmental parameters that determine how hot the conditions feel?
3. What temperature measures the combined effect of radiant heat, air temperature, and air velocity?
4. Using this combined temperature above, what temperature does the American College of Sports Medicine recommend that exercise is cancelled or postponed for heat acclimated and otherwise healthy individuals?
5. What is considered as the gold standard core body temperature measurement site?
6. True or false: Rectal temperature increases at a slower rate than oesophageal temperature and is lower than oesophageal temperature during exercise in hot conditions
7. When should you use aural/tympanic temperature to estimate core body temperature?

8. What is the commonly used equation to calculate mean skin temperature from four sites?
9. What is thermal sensation?
10. What is thermal comfort?

3.6.2 Self-check quiz answers

1. Thermal stress relates to the environmental conditions that pose a threat to thermal homeostasis, whereas thermal strain relates to the consequence of the stress e.g. a change in core body temperature caused, at least in part, by the environmental conditions.
2. Ambient temperature, humidity, air velocity, and radiant temperature.
3. Wet-bulb globe temperature.
4. 32.3°C.
5. Pulmonary arterial temperature.
6. True.
7. Never! Measuring aural temperature is attractive because it is quick, easy to do, inexpensive, and non-invasive; however, accuracy must supersede ease when deciding on a measurement site and so aural temperature should not be used even though some manufacturers provide a manual or automatic correction because of the underestimation.
8. Ramanathan (17): Mean-weighted skin temperature = (0.3 × chest skin temperature) + (0.3 × arm skin temperature) + (0.2 × thigh skin temperature) + (0.2 × lower leg skin temperature).
9. Thermal sensation (TS) quantifies the perception of temperature i.e. "what" (e.g. warm) not "how" (e.g. uncomfortable) an athlete feels.
10. Thermal comfort (TC) is a measure of "how" (e.g. uncomfortable) not "what" (e.g. warm) an athlete feels.

3.7 Practical toolkit

3.7.1 Heat stress table

Table 3.6 can be used to estimate WBGT from ambient temperature and relative humidity readings. This information can be used to help you plan training based upon the guidelines of Armstrong et al. (11).

3.7.2 Quick reference table summarising the different ways to measure heat strain

As discussed at length in this chapter, the valid and reliable measurement of core body temperature is challenging with a number of approaches used. Table 3.7 summarises the main approaches and highlights whether the answer is yes (tick) or no (cross).

TABLE 3.6 Heat stress table and recommendations for the modification or cancellation of training and non-continuous activity

Relative humidity (%)	\	Ambient temperature (°C)																														
		20	21	22	23	24	25	26	27	28	29	30	31	32	33	34	35	36	37	38	39	40	41	42	43	44	45	46	47	48	49	50
0		15	16	16	17	18	18	19	19	20	20	21	22	22	23	23	24	24	25	25	26	27	27	28	28	29	29	30	31	31	32	32
5		16	16	17	17	18	19	19	20	20	21	22	22	23	24	24	25	26	26	27	27	28	29	29	30	31	31	32	33	33	34	35
10		16	17	17	18	19	19	20	21	21	22	23	23	24	25	25	26	27	27	28	29	30	30	31	32	33	33	34	35	36	36	37
15		17	17	18	19	19	20	21	21	22	23	23	24	25	26	26	27	28	29	29	30	31	32	33	33	34	35	36	37	38	39	
20		17	18	18	19	20	20	21	22	23	23	24	24	25	26	27	28	28	29	30	31	31	32	33	34	35	36	36	37	38		
25		18	18	19	20	20	21	22	22	23	24	25	26	26	27	28	29	29	30	31	32	32	33	34	35	36	37	38				
30		18	19	20	20	21	21	22	23	24	25	26	27	27	28	29	30	30	31	32	33	34	35	36	37							
35		18	19	20	21	22	22	23	23	24	25	26	27	28	29	30	31	31	32	33	34	35	36	37	39							
40		19	20	21	21	22	23	24	24	25	26	27	28	29	30	31	32	33	34	35	36	37	38	39								
45		19	20	21	22	23	24	25	26	26	27	28	29	30	31	32	33	34	35	36	37	38	39									
50		20	21	22	23	23	24	25	26	27	28	29	30	31	32	33	34	35	36	37	38											
55		20	21	22	23	24	25	26	27	28	29	30	31	32	33	34	35	36	37	38												
60		21	22	23	24	25	26	27	28	29	30	31	32	33	34	35	36	37	38													
65		21	22	23	24	25	26	27	29	29	31	32	33	34	36	36	37	38														
70		22	23	24	25	26	27	28	29	30	31	33	34	35	36	38	39															
75		22	23	24	25	27	28	29	30	31	32	33	35	36	37	39																
80		23	24	25	26	27	28	29	30	32	33	34	35	37	38																	
85		23	24	25	26	27	29	30	31	32	34	35	36	38	39																	
90		23	24	25	26	28	29	31	32	33	35	36	37	39																		
95		24	25	26	27	28	30	31	33	34	35	37	38																			
100		24	26	27	28	29	31	32	33	35	36	38																				

Greater values all >40 °C

Recommendations from Armstrong et al. (11)

WBGT	Non-heat acclimated, unfit, high-risk individuals	Acclimated, fit, low-risk individuals
< 18.3°C	Normal activity	Normal activity
18.4 – 22.2°C	Increase the work to rest ratio and monitor fluid intake	Normal activity
22.3 – 25.6°C	Increase the work to rest ratio and decrease the total exercise duration	Normal activity but monitor fluid intake
25.7 – 27.8°C	Increase the work to rest ratio and decrease the exercise intensity and total exercise duration	Normal activity but monitor fluid intake
27.9 – 30.0°C	Increase the work to rest ratio to 1:1 and decrease the exercise intensity and total exercise duration. Limit intense exercise and monitor at-risk individuals carefully	Plan intense or prolonged exercise carefully. Monitor at-risk individuals
30.1 – 32.2°C	Cancel or stop	Limit intense exercise and exposure to heat and humidity. Keep a close eye on your athletes for sign of heat illness (See Chapter 9).
>32.3°C	Cancel exercise	Cancel exercise

TABLE 3.7 Core body temperature assessment summary

Measurement	Practical for use in the field?	Practical for use in the laboratory?	Inexpensive?	Invasive?	Acceptable agreement with pulmonary arterial temperature?	Extensive training required to use?	Well tolerated by athletes/ research participants?
Brain temperature	✗	✗	✗	✓	✓	✓	✗
Pulmonary arterial temperature	✗	✗	✗	✓	–	✓	✗
Oesophageal temperature	✗	✓/✗	✓	✓	✓	✓	✓/✗
Rectal temperature	✗	✓/✗	✓	✓	✓	✓	✓/✗
Gastrointestinal temperature	✓	✓	✗	✗	✓	✗	✓
Oral temperature	✓	✓	✓	✗	✗	✗	✓
Aural temperature	✓	✓	✓	✗	✗	✗	✓
Axillary temperature	✓	✓	✓	✗	✗	✗	✓

References

1 Glossary of terms for thermal physiology. 2nd ed. Revised by The Commission for Thermal Physiology of the International Union of Physiological Sciences (IUPS Thermal Commission). *Pflugers Arch* 1987 Nov;410(4–5):567–87.

2 Machpherson RK. The assessment of the thermal environment. A review. *Br J Ind Med* 1962 Jul;19:151–64.

3 d'Ambrosio Alfano FR, Malchaire J, Palella BI, Riccio G. WBGT index revisited after 60 years of use. *Ann Occup Hyg* 2014 Oct;58(8):955–70.

4 U.S.Army Center for Health Promotion and Preventative Medicine. Heat Stress Control and Heat Casualty Management. Aberdeen Proving Ground: USACHPPM; 2003. Report No.: TB MED 507/AFPAM 48–152.

5 Grantham J, Cheung SS, Connes P, Febbraio MA, Gaoua N, Gonzalez-Alonso J, et al. Current knowledge on playing football in hot environments. *Scand J Med Sci Sports* 2010 Oct;20 Suppl 3:161–7.

6 Mountjoy M, Alonso JM, Bergeron MF, Dvorak J, Miller S, Migliorini S, et al. Hyperthermic-related challenges in aquatics, athletics, football, tennis and triathlon. *Br J Sports Med* 2012 Sep;46(11):800–4.

7 Grimmer K, King E, Larsen T, Farquharson T, Potter A, Sharpe P, et al. Prevalence of hot weather conditions related to sports participation guidelines: a South Australian investigation. *J Sci Med Sport* 2006 May;9(1–2):72–80.

8 Cooper E, Grundstein A, Rosen A, Miles J, Ko J, Curry P. An evaluation of portable wet bulb globe temperature monitor accuracy. *J Athl Train* 2017 Dec;52(12):1161–7.

9 Liljegren JC, Carhart RA, Lawday P, Tschopp S, Sharp R. Modeling the wet bulb globe temperature using standard meteorological measurements. *J Occup Environ Hyg* 2008 Oct;5(10):645–55.

10 Roberts WO. Determining a "do not start" temperature for a marathon on the basis of adverse outcomes. *Med Sci Sports Exerc* 2010 Feb;42(2):226–32.

11 Armstrong LE, Casa DJ, Millard-Stafford M, Moran DS, Pyne SW, Roberts WO. American College of Sports Medicine position stand. Exertional heat illness during training and competition. *Med Sci Sports Exerc* 2007 Mar;39(3):556–72.

12 Malchaire J, Piette A, Kampmann B, Mehnert P, Gebhardt H, Havenith G, et al. Development and validation of the predicted heat strain model. *Ann Occup Hyg* 2001 Mar;45(2):123–35.

13 Wang F, Gao C, Kuklane K, Holmer I. Effects of various protective clothing and thermal environments on heat strain of unacclimated men: the PHS (predicted heat strain) model revisited. *Ind Health* 2013;51(3):266–74.

14 Kampmann B, Brode P, Fiala D. Physiological responses to temperature and humidity compared to the assessment by UTCI, WGBT and PHS. *Int J Biometeorol* 2012 May;56(3):505–13.

15 Fiala D, Havenith G, Brode P, Kampmann B, Jendritzky G. UTCI-Fiala multi-node model of human heat transfer and temperature regulation. *Int J Biometeorol* 2012 May;56(3):429–41.

16 International Organization for Standardization. Ergonomics – Evaluation of thermal strain by physiological measurements. Geneva: ISO; 2004. Report No.: ISO 9886.

17 Ramanathan NL. A new weighting system for mean surfacce temperature of the human body. *J Appl Physiol* 1964 May;19:531–3.

18 Robinson J, Charlton J, Seal R, Spady D, Joffres MR. Oesophageal, rectal, axillary, tympanic and pulmonary artery temperatures during cardiac surgery. *Can J Anaesth* 1998 Apr;45(4):317–23.

19 Taylor NA, Tipton MJ, Kenny GP. Considerations for the measurement of core, skin and mean body temperatures. *J Therm Biol* 2014 Dec;46:72–101.

20 Nybo L, Secher NH, Nielsen B. Inadequate heat release from the human brain during prolonged exercise with hyperthermia. *J Physiol* 2002 Dec 1;545(Pt 2):697–704.

21 Gagnon D, Lemire BB, Jay O, Kenny GP. Aural canal, esophageal, and rectal temperatures during exertional heat stress and the subsequent recovery period. *J Athl Train* 2010 Mar;45(2):157–63.

22 Mazerolle SM, Scruggs IC, Casa DJ, Burton LJ, McDermott BP, Armstrong LE, et al. Current knowledge, attitudes, and practices of certified athletic trainers regarding recognition and treatment of exertional heat stroke. *J Athl Train* 2010 Mar;45(2):170–80.

23 Miller KC, Hughes LE, Long BC, Adams WM, Casa DJ. Validity of core temperature measurements at 3 rectal depths during rest, exercise, cold-water immersion, and recovery. *J Athl Train* 2017 Apr;52(4):332–8.

24 Lee JY, Wakabayashi H, Wijayanto T, Tochihara Y. Differences in rectal temperatures measured at depths of 4–19 cm from the anal sphincter during exercise and rest. *Eur J Appl Physiol* 2010 May;109(1):73–80.

25 Ganio MS, Brown CM, Casa DJ, Becker SM, Yeargin SW, McDermott BP, et al. Validity and reliability of devices that assess body temperature during indoor exercise in the heat. *J Athl Train* 2009 Mar;44(2):124–35.

26 Teunissen LP, de HA, de Koning JJ, Daanen HA. Telemetry pill versus rectal and esophageal temperature during extreme rates of exercise-induced core temperature change. *Physiol Meas* 2012 Jun;33(6):915–24.

27 Hunt AP, Bach AJE, Borg DN, Costello JT, Stewart IB. The systematic bias of ingestible core temperature sensors requires a correction by linear regression. *Front Physiol* 2017;8:260.

28 Wilkinson DM, Carter JM, Richmond VL, Blacker SD, Rayson MP. The effect of cool water ingestion on gastrointestinal pill temperature. *Med Sci Sports Exerc* 2008 Mar;40(3):523–8.

29 Domitrovich JW, Cuddy JS, Ruby BC. Core-temperature sensor ingestion timing and measurement variability. *J Athl Train* 2010 Nov;45(6):594–600.

30 Sparling PB, Snow TK, Millard-Stafford ML. Monitoring core temperature during exercise: ingestible sensor vs. rectal thermistor. *Aviat Space Environ Med* 1993 Aug;64(8):760–3.

31 Casa DJ, Becker SM, Ganio MS, Brown CM, Yeargin SW, Roti MW, et al. Validity of devices that assess body temperature during outdoor exercise in the heat. *J Athl Train* 2007 Jul;42(3):333–42.

32 Huggins R, Glaviano N, Negishi N, Casa DJ, Hertel J. Comparison of rectal and aural core body temperature thermometry in hyperthermic, exercising individuals: a meta-analysis. *J Athl Train* 2012 May;47(3):329–38.

33 Roberts WO. Exertional heat stroke and the evolution of field care: a physician's perspective. *Temperature (Austin)* 2017;4(2):101–3.

34 Benzinger TH. Clinical temperature. New physiological basis. *JAMA* 1969 Aug 25;209(8):1200–6.

35 Brengelmann GL. Specialized brain cooling in humans? *FASEB J* 1993 Sep;7(12):1148–52.

36 Shiraki K, Sagawa S, Tajima F, Yokota A, Hashimoto M, Brengelmann GL. Independence of brain and tympanic temperatures in an unanesthetized human. *J Appl Physiol* 1988 Jul;65(1):482–6.

37 Buono MJ, Jechort A, Marques R, Smith C, Welch J. Comparison of infrared versus contact thermometry for measuring skin temperature during exercise in the heat. *Physiol Meas* 2007 Aug;28(8):855–9.

38 Tyler CJ. The effect of skin thermistor fixation method on weighted mean skin temperature. *Physiol Meas* 2011 Oct;32(10):1541–7.

39 Bach AJ, Stewart IB, Disher AE, Costello JT. A comparison between conductive and infrared devices for measuring mean skin temperature at rest, during exercise in the heat, and recovery. *PLoS One* 2015;10(2):e0117907.

40 Smith AD, Crabtree DR, Bilzon JL, Walsh NP. The validity of wireless iButtons and thermistors for human skin temperature measurement. *Physiol Meas* 2010 Jan;31(1):95–114.

41 van den Heuvel CJ, Ferguson SA, Dawson D, Gilbert SS. Comparison of digital infrared thermal imaging (DITI) with contact thermometry: pilot data from a sleep research laboratory. *Physiol Meas* 2003 Aug;24(3):717–25.

42 Fernandes AA, Amorim PR, Brito CJ, de Moura AG, Moreira DG, Costa CM, et al. Measuring skin temperature before, during and after exercise: a comparison of thermocouples and infrared thermography. *Physiol Meas* 2014 Feb;35(2):189–203.

43 Olesen BW. How many sites are necessary to estimate a mean skin temperature? In: Hales JRS, editor. Thermal Physiology. New York: Raven Press; 1984. p. 33–8.

44 Burton AC. Human calorimetry: the average temperature of the tissues of the body. *J Nut* 1935;9:261–280.

45 Stolwijk JA, Hardy JD. Partitional calorimetric studies of responses of man to thermal transients. *J Appl Physiol* 1966 May;21(3):967–77.

46 Jay O, Reardon FD, Webb P, Ducharme MB, Ramsay T, Nettlefold L, et al. Estimating changes in mean body temperature for humans during exercise using core and skin temperatures is inaccurate even with a correction factor. *J Appl Physiol (1985)* 2007 Aug;103(2):443–51.

47 Jay O, Gariepy LM, Reardon FD, Webb P, Ducharme MB, Ramsay T, et al. A three-compartment thermometry model for the improved estimation of changes in body heat content. *Am J Physiol Regul Integr Comp Physiol* 2007 Jan;292(1): R167–R175.

48 Moran DS, Shitzer A, Pandolf KB. A physiological strain index to evaluate heat stress. *Am J Physiol* 1998 Jul;275(1 Pt 2):R129–R134.

49 Tikuisis P, McLellan TM, Selkirk G. Perceptual versus physiological heat strain during exercise-heat stress. *Med Sci Sports Exerc* 2002 Sep;34(9):1454–61.

50 Gagge AP, Stolwijk JA, Saltin B. Comfort and thermal sensations and associated physiological responses during exercise at various ambient temperatures. *Environ Res* 1969 Apr;2(3):209–29.

51 Schlader ZJ, Simmons SE, Stannard SR, Mundel T. Skin temperature as a thermal controller of exercise intensity. *Eur J Appl Physiol* 2011 Aug;111(8):1631–9.

52 Gerrett N, Ouzzahra Y, Coleby S, Hobbs S, Redortier B, Voelcker T, et al. Thermal sensitivity to warmth during rest and exercise: a sex comparison. *Eur J Appl Physiol* 2014;114(7):1451–62.

53 Gagge AP, Stolwijk JA, Hardy JD. Comfort and thermal sensations and associated physiological responses at various ambient temperatures. *Environ Res* 1967 Jun;1(1):1–20.

54 ASHRAE. Handbook of Fundementals. New York: American Society of Heating, Refrigerating and Air-Conditioning Engineers; 1968.

55 ASHRAE. Standard 55-2010: Thermal environmental conditions for human occupancy. ASHRAE; 2010. Report No.: 55-2010.

56 Young AJ, Sawka MN, Epstein Y, Decristofano B, Pandolf KB. Cooling different body surfaces during upper and lower body exercise. *J Appl Physiol (1985)* 1987 Sep;63(3):1218–23.

57 Taylor NA, Allsopp NK, Parkes DG. Preferred room temperature of young vs aged males: the influence of thermal sensation, thermal comfort, and affect. *J Gerontol A Biol Sci Med Sci* 1995 Jul;50(4):M216–M221.

58 Flouris AD. Functional architecture of behavioural thermoregulation. *Eur J Appl Physiol* 2011 Jan;111(1):1–8.

59 Schlader ZJ, Simmons SE, Stannard SR, Mundel T. The independent roles of temperature and thermal perception in the control of human thermoregulatory behavior. *Physiol Behav* 2011 May 3;103(2):217–24.

60 Filingeri D, Redortier B, Hodder S, Havenith G. Thermal and tactile interactions in the perception of local skin wetness at rest and during exercise in thermo-neutral and warm environments. *Neuroscience* 2014 Jan 31;258:121–30.

61 Borg G. Psychophysical bases of perceived exertion. *Med Sci Sports Exerc* 1982;14:377–82.

4

THE EFFECT OF HIGH AMBIENT TEMPERATURES ON EXERCISE PERFORMANCE

What should you know by the end of the chapter?

As discussed in previous chapters, exercise in thermally challenging conditions increases the physiological and perceptual strain, and so it is unsurprising that such conditions can influence an athlete's ability to perform. You may have experienced this yourself if you exercise throughout the year – think back to how it felt to exercise in late winter or early spring and then compare that feeling to how it felt when you did the same route or distance in the height of summer. Thermally stressful conditions impact upon the ability to perform differently depending on the demands of the activity, and by the end of this chapter you should know:

* To what extent are the following activities affected by high levels of thermal stress?

    * Sprinting
    * Maximal voluntary force
    * Intermittent sports e.g. football
    * Middle and long distance running and cycling events

* What are some of the main theories to explain the effect that thermal stress has on the performance of these activities?

Key words, terms, and abbreviations for this chapter

Capacity test

An exercise test in which participants are asked to perform a task for as long as possible. There is no "finish line" and so these tests are sometimes referred to as "open loop" tests. Capacity tests are typically more variable than performance tests.

Central fatigue	A form of fatigue associated with changes in the concentration of neurotransmitters within the central nervous system which results in impaired exercise performance that cannot be explained by peripheral factors (e.g. decreased substrate availability).
Central governor theory	One of the theories used to explain and describe why exercise is impaired in hot conditions. It is suggested that exercise is impaired in the heat due to an anticipatory down-regulation in exercise intensity (thereby reducing endogenous heat production), in order to allow the athlete to complete the task within homeostatic limits (e.g. before you get too hot). This theory can only be observed and tested using a performance exercise test.
Critical core temperature	One of the theories used to explain and describe why exercise is impaired in hot conditions. It is suggested that once participants reach a core body temperature of ~40°C, the ability to exercise is severely compromised and exercise is stopped. This theory can only be observed and tested using a capacity exercise test.
Integrative model	A recent theory to explain the impaired exercise performance observed in hot compared to cooler conditions. The integrative governor theory suggests that exercise is regulated by competition between psychological drives and physiological protection requirements underpinned by similar basic control mechanisms, such as homeostasis and multiple negative feedback loops.
Neurotransmitter	The body's chemical messengers. Neurotransmitters are molecules that are used by the nervous system to transmit messages between neurons, or from neurons to muscles.
Performance tests	An exercise test with a fixed end-point e.g. time limit or distance target. Such tests are sometimes called closed-loop tests.
Reuptake inhibitor	A pharmacological substance that increases cerebral concentrations of a targeted neurotransmitter. For example, a noradrenaline reuptake inhibitor (reboxetine) prevents the reuptake of noradrenaline and therefore increases the amount available to act on a receptor.
Voluntary activation	The level of neural drive to muscle during exercise

Problem 4.1: What are the optimal environmental conditions for a marathon world record attempt?

You are a physiologist working for a private company attempting to set a new world record for the marathon. What would be the optimal environmental conditions for this record attempt? Why?

4.1 The effect of high ambient temperatures and humidity on sprint, intermittent, and endurance exercise performance

A moderate elevation in body temperature may be advantageous for exercise because the speed of the mechanical and metabolic processes increases by a factor of approximately two for every 10°C increase in muscle temperature (1); however, excessive elevations may impair exercise performance.

Quick question: Imagine that you are about to go for a 60 min run on a hot summer's day. Now imagine that you are going to go for the same run on a cooler spring day – how do they compare? On which occasion do you think you'd do better? For many people, the answer instinctively would be the cooler spring day, but do data from laboratory and real-world settings match this? What if rather than going for a 60 min run you were about to perform a 100 m sprint? Would your answer be the same?

Figure 4.1 shows percentage change data for a range of events – note that not all events are affected in the same way.

4.1.1 Sprint exercise performance

Single-sprint performance can be improved by warming the muscle using passive heating and/or active warm-ups. A number of potential explanations for the increase in performance with elevated muscle temperature have been proposed and these include increased phosphocreatine utilisation (3), anaerobic adenosine triphosphate turnover (4), and increased muscle fibre conduction velocity (3;5). Interestingly, warm ambient temperatures also seem to improve single-sprint performance and IAAF World Championship 100 m and 200 m sprint performances are ~2% better in hot (>25°C) conditions (2). Ball et al. (6) reported that 30 min of passive heat exposure (air temperature 30°C) increased peak power output by up to 25% compared to 30 min of temperate air exposure (19°C); however, not all studies have reported an increase in single-sprint performance in warm conditions (7). There are a number of reasons for the equivocal data (e.g. type of activity, active versus passive warming), but a key one is likely to be the effect of the ambient conditions on muscle temperature. It is not easy to passively elevate muscle temperature, and so in many cases, simply elevating ambient temperature may not have any effect on muscle temperature.

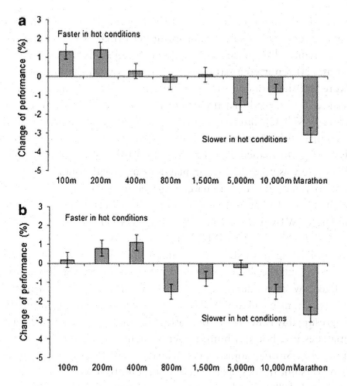

FIGURE 4.1 Mean (±95% confidence intervals) percentage change in performance observed in temperate (<25°C) and hot (>25°C) IAAF World Championship track events (1999–2011) in male (a) and female (b) athletes. Reprinted by permission from Springer Nature: Sports Medicine. Guy et al. (2). Adaptation to Hot Environmental Conditions: An Exploration of the Performance Basis, Procedures and Future Directions to Optimise Opportunities for Elite Athletes. *Sports Medicine*, 45(3): 303–11. Springer 2015.

4.1.2 Intermittent exercise and repeated sprint performance

Repeated sprint performance can be improved in hot (35°C) compared to cooler (22°C) temperatures without any noticeable differences in physiological strain when thermal strain is low (core body temperature ~37.5°C) (8); however, when thermal strain is severe (~39.5°C), repeated sprint performance is impaired (9). This impairment was observed with elevated muscle temperatures (40°C measured at a depth of 3 cm), suggesting that while elevated muscle temperatures improve explosive actions, the primary factor limiting performance in the heat is increased core body temperature. Repeated sprint performance is impaired in tennis players in hot compared to cooler conditions (~37°C versus ~22°C); however, interestingly, tennis players recovered quicker following exercise in the heat compared to cooler conditions (10). When periods long enough to allow the near complete recovery of subsequent sprint performance exist between sprints, sprint performance also appears to be only impaired if athletes are hyperthermic. Morris et al. (11) reported a strong correlation between the rate of rise in core temperature and the reduction in intermittent sprint performance while Almu-dehki et al. (12) observed that if participants remain normothermic (core body temperature = 37.3°C), intermittent sprint cycling performance is not different in 40°C compared to 24°C despite higher cardiovascular and perceptual strain. An analysis of performance data from the 2014 FIFA World Cup held in Brazil found that there was no difference in playing time, total distance covered, or the number of goals scored between matches played in low (wet-bulb globe temperature (WBGT) < 24°C at 50% relative humidity (RH); WBGT < 20°C at 75% RH), moderate (WBGT 24–28°C at 50% RH; WBGT 20–25°C at 75% RH), or high (WBGT 28–33°C at 50% RH; WBGT 25–29°C at 75% RH) environmental stress (13). Peak sprint speed was also unaffected; however, ~10% fewer sprints were completed and the distance covered at high intensity was lower under high compared to low or moderate environmental stress (~25 ± 3 m·min^1·player^{-1} versus 27 ± 2 m·min^{-1}·player^{-1}). These data suggest that elite footballers, and therefore presumably other team sport athletes, adjust their sprint activity pattern during matches in a hot and humid environment to meet the general demands of the sport (13). Similar adjustments in match activity patterns were observed in tennis players but in these players the point duration was similar between hot (34°C) and cool (19°C) conditions and the adjustment was that players took an additional ~10 s between points in the hot trial (14).

4.1.3 Prolonged exercise performance

This section will help you with Problem 4.1: What are the optimal environmental conditions for a marathon world record attempt? "You are a physiologist working for a private company attempting to set a new world record for the marathon. What would be the optimal environmental conditions for this record attempt? Why?"

The detrimental effect of hot environmental conditions on exercise performed in the laboratory is well documented and a frequently cited example of that is the data of Galloway and Maughan (15). Galloway and Maughan (15) investigated the effect of different ambient temperatures on the time taken to reach volitional exhaustion when cycling at an intensity which corresponded to 70% of the participants' individual maximal oxygen uptake. Participants took the longest to reach exhaustion at 11°C (93.5 ± 6 min) with a progressive impairment in capacity observed as temperature increased (21°C: 81.2 ± 6 min; 31°C: 51.6 ± 4 min) (Figure 4.2). Unsurprisingly, increasing the thermal stress in other ways (e.g. increasing humidity (16), increasing solar radiation (17), and decreasing air velocity (18)) also impairs exercise capacity in a progressive manner (Figure 4.2). Compared to the optimal condition, increases in thermal stress impair exercise capacity by between 7% and 54% with a mean impairment of approximately 30% (15–18).

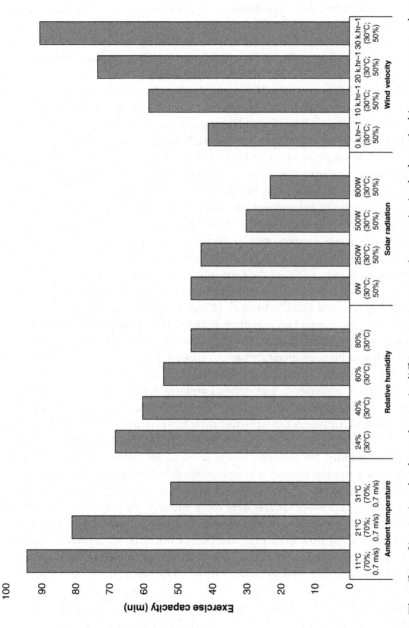

FIGURE 4.2 The effect of increasing the thermal stress in different ways on exercise capacity in the heat. Ambient temperature data (RH and wind velocity) from Galloway and Maughan (15); RH data (ambient temperature) from Maughan et al. (16); solar radiation data (ambient temperature; RH) from Otani et al. (17); wind velocity data (ambient temperature and RH) from Otani et al. (18).

Due to the open-loop nature of a capacity test (i.e. there is no "finish line"), such tests are typically more variable than performance tests (closed-loop tests with a fixed end e.g. time limit or distance target), and the magnitude of changes observed tends to be larger. The difference in performance tests in hot compared to cooler conditions is smaller than the difference in capacity tests but impairments are still observed. For example, Tyler et al. (19) observed that ~10% less distance was ran during a 15 min time trial in hot (~31°C) compared to moderate (~14°C) conditions (3,574 ± 414 m versus 3,210 ± 531 m).

Laboratory data are often collected on sub-elite ("recreationally active") participants and the magnitude of impairment observed in this population appears larger than that observed in elite athletes e.g. the impairment observed in IAAF World Championship events over 5,000 m undertaken in hot conditions (>25°C) is ~2% (2). The negative effect of high ambient temperatures on IAAF World Championship performances is greatest in the marathon (3.1% for males and 2.7% for females) (2) and this is likely to be due to the metabolic demands of the event. Core body and ambient temperatures are independent of one another over a range called the "prescriptive" zone (20); however, as the metabolic rate increases, this range narrows, and so climatic conditions have a greater effect on metabolically demanding activities. Competitive marathon runners run at a pace approximately ~75% of their maximal oxygen uptake for over 2 h (21) and so it is unsurprising that impairments in marathon performance in the heat are regularly reported (22;23). El et al. (22) investigated the effects of different environmental parameters on marathon performance at six of the world's most prestigious races (Berlin, Boston, Chicago, London, New York, and Paris) and observed that ambient temperature had the greatest impact and humidity had the second biggest impact (both greater than the dew point, atmospheric pressure, and atmospheric pollutants). The optimal ambient temperature was calculated as ~3.8°C for elite male runners and ~9.9°C for elite female runners and slightly warmer for slower runners (first quartile: male 6.0°C; female: 6.9°C; third quartile: male: 7.4°C; female: 7.4°C) (22). Ely et al. (22) also investigated the effect of ambient temperature on performances at seven major marathons and observed that the fastest runners slowed as temperatures increased with male and female runners running approximately 4.3% and 5.6% slower in 20–25°C compared to 5–10°C (WBGT). Slower runners were more effected that faster ones with runners in the 300th percentile running approximately 21% slower (23) (Figure 4.3). Not only does an increase in thermal stress slow runners down, it can cause them to stop altogether with the percentage of elite athletes completing the marathon at the Olympic games dropping from ~79% to ~54% when the ambient temperature exceeds 25°C (24).

Prolonged cycling performance may be less affected by high ambient temperatures than running. Chan et al. (25) studied the effects of a hot environment (31°C; 76% RH) on simulated duathlon of sorts (40 km cycling followed by 10 km running) in triathletes. Compared to moderate conditions (22°C; 76% RH), the overall performance time was slower in the heat but interestingly this

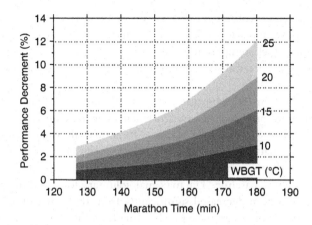

FIGURE 4.3 Nomogram showing the relationship between thermal stress (WBGT) and marathon performance decrement. Modified from (23).

was because the run was slower (51 ± 4 min versus 59 ± 5 min) – there were no differences in the cycling time. The difference is likely to be due to a number of factors, such as running having a greater endogenous heat production for a given metabolic rate and exposing athletes to lower airflow speeds than cycling. With a representative airflow (~32 km h^{-1}), cycling power output and 40 km cycling performance are similar in 17°C, 22°C, and 27°C dry air temperature conditions but impaired in 32°C (26).

4.2 The effect of high ambient temperatures and humidity on neuromuscular performance

As mentioned, thermal stress can impair exercise performance if it results in thermal strain. Hyperthermia may have a direct effect upon the central nervous system by reducing the drive to the motorneuron pool (27) when core body temperatures are elevated (28). Nybo and Nielsen (28) asked their participants to cycle to exhaustion (at an intensity corresponding to 60% of the participants' maximal oxygen uptake) in hot (40°C) and temperate (18°C) conditions. Participants reached core temperatures of ~40°C in the hot trial and prematurely terminated exercise after ~50 min but in the cooler conditions, core temperature plateaued at ~38°C and participants were able to complete the 1 h of exercise. Maximal voluntary force production and the percentage of voluntary activation in the exercised muscle groups (knee extensors) were reduced following the exercise bout to a greater extent in the hot, compared to cooler, trial. There was a reduction in maximal *voluntary* force but the capability of the muscle was not different between the hot and cool trials. An electrical stimulation was applied to the femoral nerve to maximally recruit the muscle fibres of the quadriceps (and therefore produce maximal *involuntary* force) and what this showed was that, despite reaching volitional exhaustion in the hot trials, the capacity for the muscle to generate force was unaffected by the ambient conditions or the elevated core and muscle temperatures observed in the hot trials. In other words, the superimposed electrical stimulation induced the same overall force in both conditions.

Nybo and Nielsen (28) observed reduced voluntary force production when hyperthermic with pre- and post-measurements but the reduction in voluntary force production appears to be progressive. Morrison et al. (29) asked participants to perform maximal voluntary isometric contractions at 0.5°C core temperature intervals as they were passively warmed from ~37.5°C to ~39.5°C and then cooled back down to baseline. The maximal voluntary force and the percentage of voluntary activation decreased significantly from the start to the end of the passive warming bout but returned to baseline levels at the end of the cooling bout in a progressive manner.

4.3 Why is prolonged exercise performance impaired in thermally challenging conditions?

The aetiology of the premature fatigue often observed during exercise is likely to involve a complex interaction between the cardiovascular, muscular, and central nervous systems. The impaired ability to perform is observed in high ambient temperatures, high humidity, and when airflow is reduced (see Chapter 3 for more information on how different aspects of the environmental conditions can interact to alter the thermal stress faced).

4.3.1 The critical core temperature hypothesis

Observations that participants consistently terminate fixed-intensity exercise at core temperatures of ~40°C regardless of acclimation status (30) or initial core temperature (31) led to the hypothesis that there is a critical body temperature that limits the ability to exercise (or work) in the heat (30). The interest in the possible existence of a critical core temperature stemmed largely from a study investigating the effect of heat acclimation on the human circulatory and thermoregulatory response to exercise in a hot environment (30). Nielsen et al. (30) reported that, although exercise capacity time almost doubled following a 9–12 day heat acclimation protocol, voluntary exhaustion occurred consistently at an oesophageal temperature of ~39.7°C. At the point of exhaustion, there were no reductions in cardiac output, muscle blood flow, or skin blood flow and there was no lack of substrate or any accumulation of any substance traditionally thought to cause fatigue such as lactate or potassium ions and therefore the authors proposed the concept of exercise-limiting hyperthermia. Further support for the idea of a critical cut-off core body temperature was provided by Gonzalez-Alonso and colleagues (31), who asked participants to cycle to volitional exhaustion on three occasions with manipulated starting core body temperatures of ~36°C (cool), ~37°C (control), and ~38°C (warm). Participants completed 63 ± 3, 46 ± 3, and 28 ± 2 min in the cool, control, and hot trials, respectively, but despite the marked differences in capacity time, all trials were voluntarily terminated at remarkably consistent core body temperatures: 40.1 ± 0.1°C, 40.2 ± 0.1°C, and 40.1 ± 0.1°C (31).

4.3.2 The central governor theory and anticipatory thermoregulation

The critical core temperature theory proposes that exercise is terminated due to the attainment of a high core body temperature, which results in a catastrophic physiological event (i.e. the stopping of exercise); however, it has been shown that, during self-paced exercise, a down-regulation of running speed and power output occurs long before such core body temperatures are reached. For example, Tucker et al. (32) reported that although rectal temperatures were the same for the first 15 km (75%) of a 20 km cycling time trial in hot (35°C) and cool (15°C) conditions, work rate and muscle recruitment were down-regulated in the hot conditions within the first 30% of the trial.

It has been proposed that this down-regulation is to allow athletes to be able to complete the task within homeostatic limits (i.e. before they get too hot). Tatterson et al. (33) reported that 30 min cycling time-trial performance was impaired in hot (32°C) compared to moderate (23°C) conditions but despite the differences in ambient conditions and total work done, participants finished the time trial at near identical core temperatures (39.2 ± 0.2 versus 39.0 ± 0.1°C). Marino et al. (34) provided further support for the anticipatory mechanism when comparing Caucasian and African runners. Each group ran for 30 min submaximally prior to an 8 km time trial in hot (35°C) conditions. Rectal temperatures were similar at the end of the 30 min submaximal phase (~38.4°C) and at the end of the self-paced performance test (~39.3°C), the African runners ran faster than the Caucasian runners, completing the time trial about 3 min quicker (30 ± 2 versus 33 ± 2 min). The rate at which core temperature rose was similar in the two groups (2.2 versus 3.2°C·h^{1}) despite the difference in pace suggesting that the Caucasian athletes selected a pace that allowed them to complete the task – if they had set off any quicker they may have had to slow down or stop prior to completing the test. The slower pace was selected immediately during the time trial despite similar rectal temperatures between the groups and Marino et al. (34) proposed that rather than being limited by the attainment of a critically high temperature, exercise performance is determined by the rate at which body temperature increases.

Evidence for the role of the central nervous system in the down-regulation of skeletal muscle recruitment during exercise-induced hyperthermia has been provided by electrical stimulation studies. By superimposing an electrical stimulation on top of a voluntary contraction and calculating the ratio between the voluntary and evoked contractions, the level of central activation can be evaluated (28). As previously discussed, Morrison et al. (35) reported a gradual reduction in voluntary activation percentage when participants were passively warmed from rectal temperatures of ~37.5°C to temperatures of ~39.5°C. The activation percentage was restored when the internal temperatures returned to the initial values, indicating a gradual reduction in central nervous system drive as hyperthermia develops.

4.3.2.1 The critical core temperature hypothesis "versus" the central governor theory and anticipatory thermoregulation

The central governor theory and critical core temperature models are often reported as being opposing viewpoints; however, they are in fact very similar in their main theme of preventing the development of a high core temperature and the onset of potentially fatal heat illness. The obtainment of a high core temperature results in the termination of exercise in tests of fixed intensity (31;36), whereas the central governor theory highlights that in self-paced activity the work rate is down-regulated well before a high core temperature is reached (33;34). The differences reported appear to exist largely as a result of the exercise model investigated. The critical core temperature model can only be observed in steady-state, exercise capacity tests, whereas the central governor model can only be observed in self-paced performance tests. It is clear that the development of a high core body temperature plays a role in limiting exercise performed in the heat but it is also clear that there are weaknesses with these two highly cited theories. The critical core temperature and central fatigue hypotheses provide models from which to gain a greater understanding of the reasons limiting performance but they do not describe how hyperthermia ultimately limits exercise.

4.3.3 The central fatigue theory

Many researchers have suggested that the fatigue observed due to hyperthermia may occur due to alterations in cerebral neurotransmitter activity and concentrations of serotonin and dopamine (37). Serotonin is a monoamine neurotransmitter linked to the augmentation of lethargy and the loss of drive, and so it was suggested that fatigue may occur as a result of increased serotonin activity in the brain. Serotonin formed the basis of the original central fatigue hypothesis (38); however, the administration of serotonin receptor antagonists (which should increase cerebral serotonin concentrations) had no effect on running capacity (39) or performance in hot conditions (35°C) (40) and so other candidates have received attention. One such candidate is dopamine which is linked with feelings of arousal and motivation (41). Cerebral dopamine concentrations can be elevated by administering a dopamine reuptake inhibitor such as those prescribed as antidepressants. Acute administration of both bupropion (which inhibits the reuptake of dopamine and noradrenaline in the brain meaning that concentrations of both remain elevated), and methylphenidate (Ritalin – which elevates dopamine only) has no effect on cycling performance in ambient conditions of 18°C but significantly improves performance in hot (30°C) conditions (42;43). Watson et al. (43) reported that bupropion improved cycling performance by ~9% in the heat and that seven of the nine participants achieved rectal temperatures of ≥40°C in the bupropion trial compared to only two in the control trial. Despite the higher physiological strain and exercise intensity, perceived strain was not altered suggesting that the administration of the pharmacological agent may have overridden inhibitory signals and enabled the participants to cycle faster.

Elevating noradrenaline alone by administering a noradrenaline reuptake inhibitor (reboxetine) impairs cycling performance in 18°C (by ~10%) and 30°C (by ~20%) conditions (44), whereas cycling performance is improved by ~16% when elevating dopamine concentrations (following the administration of Ritalin) in warm conditions (30°C). Elevating dopamine had no effect on performance in moderate (18°C) trials (42). These data in combination suggest that dopamine plays a dominant role in thermoregulation and the enhancement of exercise in a hot environment (Figure 4.4).

4.3.4 Integrative model

As highlighted, there are a number of mechanisms and theories used to explain or describe the premature fatigue observed in hot compared to cooler conditions. To consider them in isolation is a reductionist approach as they are all likely to play a role (probably with other, yet to be identified, mechanisms) and so a "higher order", integrative model has been proposed by St Clair Gibson et al. (46). The integrative governor theory suggests that exercise is regulated by competition between psychological drives and physiological protection

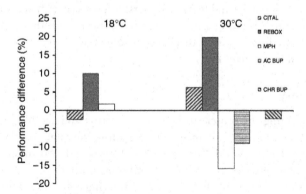

FIGURE 4.4 The effects of various pharmacological manipulations in normal and high ambient temperatures on cycling performance. CITAL = citalopram; REBOX = reboxetine; MPH = methylphenidate; AC BUP = acute bupropion; CHR BUP = chronic bupropion. Figure reproduced from Meeusen and Roelands (45) with permission. 2010 John Wiley & Sons A/S.

requirements underpinned by similar basic control mechanisms such as homeo-stasis and multiple negative feedback loops (46). It is clear that the reasons for the premature termination of exercise in hot compared to temperate environments are multifaceted and complex and so an integrated model is appropriate; how-ever, it is likely that the current integrated model will evolve as new insights are made.

Problem 4.1 revisited: What are the optimal environmental conditions for a marathon world record attempt?

You are a physiologist working for a private company attempting to set a new world record for the marathon. What would be the optimal environmental conditions for this record attempt? Why?

By now, you should be aware that the marathon running performance is im-paired in hot conditions (if not, reread Section 4.1.3!). Guy et al. reported that it is the IAAF World Championship marathon which is ~3% slower in the heat (2) and Ely et al. (22) reported that male and female runners run approximately ~5% slower at 20–25°C compared to 5–10°C (WBGT). Slower runners are more affected than faster ones (23) but this does not apply to this question because you are part of a world record attempt. The current marathon world records are 2:01:39 (set by Eliud Kipchoge of Kenya at the 2018 Berlin Marathon) and 2:17:01 (set by Mary Keitany on 23 April 2017 at the London Marathon) for male and female runners, respectively (Paula Radcliffe hold the world record for the mixed-gender marathon – 2:15:25). These times barely make it on to the nomo-gram produced by Ely et al. (23), but the nomogram still suggests that if WBGT increases above 10°C performance, it is likely to be impaired by 1–2%.

El et al. (22) calculated the optimal marathon running temperature as ~3.8°C and ~9.9°C for elite male and female runners, respectively (22) and so to make a reasonable attempt at setting a new marathon world record, these temperatures should be planned for ensuring that there is some airflow (tailwind rather than headwind) and low radiant heat.

4.4 Summary

Although warming the muscle using passive heating and active warm-ups can improve single-sprint performance, data regarding the effect on thermal stress are equivocal. IAAF World Championship 100 m and 200 m sprint perfor-mances are ~2% better in hot (>25°C) conditions (2) but not all studies report improvements (7). This is likely to be due to differing effects of thermal stress on muscle temperature – simply being in a warm climate will not warm the muscle. There is a strong relationship between the rate of rise in core temperature and the reduction in intermittent sprint performance (11) and such performance appears to be improved in warm conditions as long as thermal strain is low (8). Unlike shorter duration events, prolonged exercise (15) and neuromuscular performance (28) are consistently impaired in hot laboratory conditions. The impairment in prolonged exercise is observed in real-world settings too, with the greatest impairments observed in the longest events (2).

Exercise performance and capacity are regularly impaired in hot compared to moderate conditions but the reasons are not fully understood. During fixed-intensity laboratory protocols, exercise capacity is voluntarily terminated at a core body temperature of ~40°C but temperatures can be tolerated well by well-motivated athletes. In performance studies, self-selected intensity is reduced prior to the obtainment of high internal temperatures suggesting that an anticipatory down-regulation allows for the task to be completed within homeostatic limits (32;47). Fatigue in the heat does not occur as a result of many peripherally located causes of fatigue in temperate conditions (30) and therefore the suggestion that it is a centrally regulated fatigue appears to be the most plausible proposal. Data suggest that cerebral dopamine concentrations play a dominant role in the regulation of exercise performance and adherence in hot environmental conditions (42;44).

4.5 Self-check quiz

Anecdotally, you are probably well aware that exercising in hot conditions feels different to exercising in cooler conditions and that depending on what activity you are undertaking the exercise may feel easier or harder. At the start of the chapter, we highlighted that you should know the following by this point:

- To what extent are the following activities affected by high levels of thermal stress?
  - Sprinting
  - Maximal voluntary force
  - Intermittent sports e.g. football
  - Middle- and long-distance events
- What are some of the main theories to explain the effect that thermal stress has on the performance of these activities?

The self-check quiz below will help you see whether the learning objectives of this chapter have been achieved. Before looking at the answers, if you are stuck on any question, try looking back at the relevant section. For help with questions 1–4, take another look at Section 4.1; for help with questions 5 and 6, take another look at Section 4.2; and if you are stuck on questions 7–10, Section 4.3 will help.

4.5.1 Self-check quiz questions

1. What types of exercise are most affected by hot conditions?
2. What types of exercise are least affected by hot conditions?
3. Intermittent-sprint performance can be improved by warmer conditions unless what occurs?

4. What is the optimal temperature for elite marathon running according to the data of El et al. (22)?
5. What is the relationship between hyperthermia and maximal voluntary force production?
6. Why did Nybo and Nielsen (among others) superimpose an electrical twitch onto the femoral nerve while their participants performed a maximal voluntary contraction? What data does this technique yield that helps explain impaired exercise performance seen in hot conditions?
7. What temperature is often referred to as a "critical core body temperature"?
8. What are the names of the two models that involve an anticipatory reduction in self-selected exercise intensity to describe why exercise performance is impaired in the heat?
9. What exercise test (capacity or time-trial) can be used to test the critical core temperature model?
10. What neurotransmitter is likely to play a key role in regulating exercise performance in hot conditions?

4.5.2 Self-check quiz answers

1. Long-duration events e.g. marathon running. Marathon performance is impaired by ~3.1% in elite males and by ~2.7% in elite females (2).
2. Short-duration, high-intensity exercise. For example, IAAF World Championship 100 m and 200 m sprint performances are ~2% better in hot (>25°C) compared to cooler (<25°C) conditions (2).
3. Repeated sprint performance is impaired when the magnitude of thermal strain is severe (~39.5°C) (14).
4. ~3.8°C for elite male runners and ~9.9°C for elite female runners.
5. Linear. Maximal voluntary force is reduced as core body temperature increases (and can be restored as core body temperature reduces).
6. Superimposing the twitch allows the researchers to see where the muscle is being fully activated voluntarily. If the twitch results in the muscle producing more force than it was during the contraction, it shows that the muscle is capable of producing higher forces and that there is some sort of inhibition.
7. ~40°C.
8. The central governor and integrative models.
9. Capacity.
10. Dopamine.

References

1 Belehradek J. Physiological aspects of heat and cold. *Annu Rev Physiol* 1957;19:59–82.
2 Guy JH, Deakin GB, Edwards AM, Miller CM, Pyne DB. Adaptation to hot environmental conditions: an exploration of the performance basis, procedures and future directions to optimise opportunities for elite athletes. *Sports Med* 2015 Mar;45(3):303–11.

3 Gray SR, De VG, Nimmo MA, Farina D, Ferguson RA. Skeletal muscle ATP turnover and muscle fiber conduction velocity are elevated at higher muscle temperatures during maximal power output development in humans. *Am J Physiol Regul Integr Comp Physiol* 2006 Feb;290(2):R376–R382.

4 Febbraio MA, Carey MF, Snow RJ, Stathis CG, Hargreaves M. Influence of elevated muscle temperature on metabolism during intense, dynamic exercise. *Am J Physiol* 1996 Nov;271(5 Pt 2):R1251–R1255.

5 Farina D, Arendt-Nielsen L, Graven-Nielsen T. Effect of temperature on spike-triggered average torque and electrophysiological properties of low-threshold motor units. *J Appl Physiol (1985)* 2005 Jul;99(1):197–203.

6 Ball D, Burrows C, Sargeant AJ. Human power output during repeated sprint cycle exercise: the influence of thermal stress. *Eur J Appl Physiol Occup Physiol* 1999 Mar;79(4):360–6.

7 Backx K, McNaughton L, Crickmore L, Palmer G, Carlisle A. Effects of differing heat and humidity on the performance and recovery from multiple high intensity, intermittent exercise bouts. *Int J Sports Med* 2000 Aug;21(6):400–5.

8 Falk B, Radom-Isaac S, Hoffmann JR, Wang Y, Yarom Y, Magazanik A, et al. The effect of heat exposure on performance of and recovery from high-intensity, intermittent exercise. *Int J Sports Med* 1998 Jan;19(1):1–6.

9 Drust B, Rasmussen P, Mohr M, Nielsen B, Nybo L. Elevations in core and muscle temperature impairs repeated sprint performance. *Acta Physiol Scand* 2005 Feb;183(2):181–90.

10 Girard O, Christian RJ, Racinais S, Periard JD. Heat stress does not exacerbate tennis-induced alterations in physical performance. *Br J Sports Med* 2014 Apr;48 Suppl 1:i39–i44.

11 Morris JG, Nevill ME, Boobis LH, Macdonald IA, Williams C. Muscle metabolism, temperature, and function during prolonged, intermittent, high-intensity running in air temperatures of 33 degrees and 17 degrees C. *Int J Sports Med* 2005 Dec;26(10):805–14.

12 Almudehki F, Girard O, Grantham J, Racinais S. Hot ambient conditions do not alter intermittent cycling sprint performance. *J Sci Med Sport* 2012 Mar;15(2):148–52.

13 Nassis GP, Brito J, Dvorak J, Chalabi H, Racinais S. The association of environmental heat stress with performance: analysis of the 2014 FIFA World Cup Brazil. *Br J Sports Med* 2015 May;49(9):609–13.

14 Periard JD, Racinais S, Knez WL, Herrera CP, Christian RJ, Girard O. Thermal, physiological and perceptual strain mediate alterations in match-play tennis under heat stress. *Br J Sports Med* 2014 Apr;48 Suppl 1:i32–i38.

15 Galloway SDR, Maughan RJ. Effects of ambient temperature on the capacity to perform prolonged exercise in man. *Med Sci Sports Exerc* 1997;29:1240–9.

16 Maughan RJ, Otani H, Watson P. Influence of relative humidity on prolonged exercise capacity in a warm environment. *Eur J Appl Physiol* 2012 Jun;112(6):2313–21.

17 Otani H, Kaya M, Tamaki A, Watson P, Maughan RJ. Effects of solar radiation on endurance exercise capacity in a hot environment. *Eur J Appl Physiol* 2016 Apr;116(4):769–79.

18 Otani H, Kaya M, Tamaki A, Watson P, Maughan RJ. Air velocity influences thermoregulation and endurance exercise capacity in the heat. *Appl Physiol Nutr Metab* 2018 Feb;43(2):131–8.

19 Tyler C, Sunderland C. The effect of ambient temperature on the reliability of a preloaded treadmill time-trial. *Int J Sports Med* 2008 Oct;29(10):812–6.

20 Lind AR. A physiological criterion for setting thermal environmental limits for everyday work. *J Appl Physiol* 1963 Jan;18:51–6.

21 Maughan RJ, Leiper JB. Aerobic capacity and fractional utilisation of aerobic capacity in elite and non-elite male and female marathon runners. *Eur J Appl Physiol Occup Physiol* 1983;52(1):80–7.

22 El HN, Tafflet M, Berthelot G, Tolaini J, Marc A, Guillaume M, et al. Impact of environmental parameters on marathon running performance. *PLoS One* 2012;7(5):e37407.

23 Ely MR, Cheuvront SN, Roberts WO, Montain SJ. Impact of weather on marathon-running performance. *Med Sci Sports Exerc* 2007 Mar;39(3):487–93.

24 Martin DE, Gynn RWH. The Olympic marathon. Champaign, IL: Human Kinetics; 2000.

25 Chan KO, Wong SH, Chen YJ. Effects of a hot environment on simulated cycling and running performance in triathletes. *J Sports Med Phys Fitness* 2008 Jun;48(2):149–57.

26 Peiffer JJ, Abbiss CR. Influence of environmental temperature on 40 km cycling time-trial performance. *Int J Sports Physiol Perform* 2011 Jun;6(2):208–20.

27 Gandevia SC. Spinal and supraspinal factors in human muscle fatigue. Physiol Rev 2001 Oct;81(4):1725–89.

28 Nybo L, Nielsen B. Hyperthermia and central fatigue during prolonged exercise in humans. *J Appl Physiol* 2001 Sep;91(3):1055–60.

29 Morrison S, Sleivert GG, Cheung SS. Passive hyperthermia reduces voluntary activation and isometric force production. *Eur J Appl Physiol* 2004 May;91(5–6):729–36.

30 Nielsen B, Hales JR, Strange S, Christensen NJ, Warberg J, Saltin B. Human circulatory and thermoregulatory adaptations with heat acclimation and exercise in a hot, dry environment. *J Physiol* 1993 Jan;460:467–85.

31 Gonzalez-Alonso J, Teller C, Andersen SL, Jensen FB, Hyldig T, Nielsen B. Influence of body temperature on the development of fatigue during prolonged exercise in the heat. *J Appl Physiol* 1999 Mar;86(3):1032–9.

32 Tucker R, Rauch L, Harley YX, Noakes TD. Impaired exercise performance in the heat is associated with an anticipatory reduction in skeletal muscle recruitment. *Pflugers Arch* 2004 Jul;448(4):422–30.

33 Tatterson AJ, Hahn AG, Martin DT, Febbraio MA. Effects of heat stress on physiological responses and exercise performance in elite cyclists. *J Sci Med Sport* 2000 Jun;3(2):186–93.

34 Marino FE, Lambert MI, Noakes TD. Superior performance of African runners in warm humid but not in cool environmental conditions. *J Appl Physiol* 2004;96(1):124–30.

35 Morrison SA, Cheung S, Cotter JD. Importance of airflow for physiologic and ergogenic effects of precooling. *J Athl Train* 2014 Sep;49(5):632–9.

36 Walters TJ, Ryan KL, Tate LM, Mason PA. Exercise in the heat is limited by a critical internal temperature. *J Appl Physiol* 2000 Aug;89(2):799–806.

37 Meeusen R, Watson P, Hasegawa H, Roelands B, Piacentini MF. Central fatigue: the serotonin hypothesis and beyond. *Sports Med* 2006;36(10):881–909.

38 Newsholme EA, Blomstrand E. Tryptophan, 5-hydroxytryptamine and a possible explanation for central fatigue. *Adv Exp Med Biol* 1995;384:315–20.

39 Pannier JL, Bouckaert JJ, Lefebvre RA. The antiserotonin agent pizotifen does not increase endurance performance in humans. *Eur J Appl Physiol Occup Physiol* 1995;72(1–2):175–8.

40 Strachan AT, Leiper JB, Maughan RJ. Serotonin2C receptor blockade and thermoregulation during exercise in the heat. *Med Sci Sports Exerc* 2005 Mar;37(3):389–94.

41 Chaouloff F. Physical exercise and brain monoamines: a review. *Acta Physiol Scand* 1989 Sep;137(1):1–13.

42 Roelands B, Hasegawa H, Watson P, Piacentini MF, Buyse L, De SG, et al. The effects of acute dopamine reuptake inhibition on performance. *Med Sci Sports Exerc* 2008 May;40(5):879–85.

43 Watson P, Hasegawa H, Roelands B, Piacentini MF, Looverie R, Meeusen R. Acute dopamine/noradrenaline reuptake inhibition enhances human exercise performance in warm, but not in temperate conditions. *J Physiol* 2005 Jun 15;565(Pt 3):873–83.

44 Roelands B, Goekint M, Heyman E, Piacentini MF, Watson P, Hasegawa H, et al. Acute norepinephrine reuptake inhibition decreases performance in normal and high ambient temperature. *J Appl Physiol* 2008 Jul;105(1):206–12.

45 Meeusen R, Roelands B. Central fatigue and neurotransmitters, can thermoregulation be manipulated? *Scand J Med Sci Sports* 2010 Oct;20 Suppl 3:19–28.

46 St Clair Gibson A, Swart J, Tucker R. The interaction of psychological and physiological homeostatic drives and role of general control principles in the regulation of physiological systems, exercise and the fatigue process – the integrative governor theory. *Eur J Sport Sci* 2018 Feb;18(1):25–36.

47 Noakes TD, St Clair GA. Logical limitations to the "catastrophe" models of fatigue during exercise in humans. *Br J Sports Med* 2004;38(5):648–9.

5

THE EFFECT OF HIGH AMBIENT TEMPERATURES ON COGNITIVE FUNCTION

What should you know by the end of the chapter?

While the effects of thermal stress and strain on exercise performance are well documented, less attention has been paid to the effects of hyperthermia and thermal stress on cognitive performance. This is somewhat surprising because successful sporting performance requires the athlete to be proficient in a number of areas of cognitive function (e.g. efficient and accurate decision-making). This chapter will summarise the current state of knowledge regarding cognitive performance in hot conditions. By the end of the chapter you should know:

- What is cognitive function and what are its subcomponents?
- How is cognitive function assessed?
- How is cognitive function affected by hyperthermia?
- Why is cognitive function affected by hyperthermia?
- What other factors can affect the cognitive function of athletes competing in hot conditions?

Key terms for this chapter

Alpha waves	Low-frequency brainwaves (frequency = 8–13 Hz). Increases in alpha wave activity are linked to decreased arousal and are most apparent during sleep or periods when the participant has their eyes closed.
Arousal	A physiological and psychological state of being alert, awake, and attentive.

Attention	One of the five main areas of cognitive function. Attention is the ability to focus on relevant information while ignoring irrelevant information.
Beta waves	High-frequency brainwaves (frequency = 13–30 Hz). Decreases in beta wave activity is linked to decreased arousal and therefore potentially impaired cognitive function.
Cognitive function	A measure of the accuracy and efficiency of cortical and subcortical processes in detecting, identifying, and responding to external stimuli. The five main areas of cognitive function are:

1 Executive function (See Executive function)
2 Memory (see Memory)
3 Attention (see Attention)
4 Social and emotional cognition (see Social and emotional cognition)
5 Psychomotor speed (see Psychomotor speed)

Electroencephalography (EEG)	A test that detects electrical activity in the brain using electrodes attached to the scalp.
Executive function	One of the five main areas of cognitive function. Executive function is the ability to make high-level and complex decisions.
Frontal lobe	Part of the brain which is located at the front and involved in important cognitive skills such as working memory tasks.
Memory	One of the five main areas of cognitive function. Memory is the ability to retain information.
Occipital lobe	Located at the rear, this region of the brain is the visual processing centre of the brain.
Parietal lobe	This region of the brain receives and processes sensory information.
Psychomotor speed	One of the five main areas of cognitive function. Psychomotor speed is the ability to detect and respond to an appropriate stimulus.
Social and emotional cognition	One of the five main areas of cognitive function. Social and emotional cognition is the ability to respond to emotion-laden stimuli.

| Theta waves | Low-frequency brainwaves (frequency = 3–8 Hz). Increases in theta wave activity indicate increases in mental workload and cognitive fatigue. |

Problem 5.1. How can you minimise the effect of exercise in the heat on the cognitive function of your athlete?

You are the coach of an elite field hockey player who is an integral member of the team but whose decision-making declines markedly when the level of thermal stress is high. Field hockey allows for rolling substitutions and so it is typical for players to routinely spend a few minutes off the pitch between bouts of high-intensity exercise. What intervention(s) could you try in order to minimise the impairment in decision-making that was previously observed? In order to answer this problem you will need to consider what might explain the impairment.

5.1 Cognitive function

5.1.1 What is cognitive function?

Quick question: Before we move on, how would you define cognitive function? What is it?

Cognitive function is a measure of the accuracy and efficiency of cortical and subcortical processes in detecting, identifying, and responding to internal and external stimuli. If you imagine that you are playing a game of football, there is a lot of information that you are provided with. Some of the information may be very relevant (e.g. the flight of the ball towards you), some might be potentially relevant (e.g. the position of your full back who might be a suitable teammate to pass to if the ball makes it you), and some may have no real relevance at all (e.g. the two fans who are leaving their seat just before half-time to beat the queues at the bar); in order to be successful, you need to be able to react to and focus on the relevant information efficiently and accurately. In order to do this, you will need to demonstrate skilled cognitive function – an umbrella term used to describe a number of functions that usually operate in parallel with one another. The five areas of cognitive function (and their subdomains) that have received the most attention are as follows (although there is some overlap between them):

- Executive function: The ability to make high-level and complex decisions. There are four main subdomains:

    1 Mental flexibility – can you adapt your thinking and behaviour?
    2 Working memory – can you adopt an effective strategy?
    3 Planning – are you strategic when solving a problem?
    4 Response inhibition – can you stop yourself from performing an inappropriate or incorrect action?

- Memory: The ability to retain information over short or prolonged periods of time (short-term and long-term memory, respectively). There are three main subdomains:

  1 Episodic memory – can you associate an event with a specific time or place?
  2 Recognition memory – can you effectively recognise the stimulus presented?
  3 Working memory – can you effectively hold and manipulate the information stored?

- Attention: The ability to focus on relevant information and ignore the irrelevant information. Attention has one main subdomain:

  1 Sustained attention – can you maintain appropriate selective attention for a prolonged period of time?

- Psychomotor speed: The ability to detect and respond to an appropriate stimulus. Often this is assessed using either a simple (one stimulus) or choice (multiple stimuli) reaction time test.
- Social and emotional cognition: The ability to respond to emotion-laden stimuli. It can be broken down in to two subdomains:

  1 Emotion recognition – can you accurately identify emotions in facial expressions?
  2 Emotional bias – how do you process information with positive or negative social connotations?

5.1.2 How is cognitive function assessed?

Cognitive function is often tested using a battery of tests that assess behaviour (e.g. speed and accuracy of response) to infer the effectiveness of cognitive operations such as working memory. Cognitive function tests are often computer or tablet based and vary in complexity – the range of complexity is to allow various functions to be assessed and ensure that the test is population specific e.g. a healthy, well-trained athlete would be expected to have a higher baseline than an elderly individual with an illness such as dementia and so would require a more challenging test battery. The test used is determined by the aspect of cognitive function that is to be tested; however, some tests can provide information on a number of domains. Commonly used cognitive function tests include the paired associates learning test, the simple reaction time test, and the Stroop test but the range of tests used is vast (Figure 5.1).

As with all testing, in order to accurately assess cognitive function, effective pretrial standardisation, calibration, and familiarisation are required. In addition to controls mentioned previously, because the tests are predominantly computer based, there are extra considerations to be aware of e.g. what is the lag time between response (e.g. mouse click, keyboard tap, touchscreen contact) and

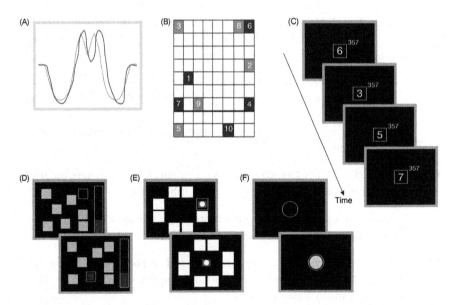

FIGURE 5.1 Examples of computer-based cognitive function tests assessing (A) fine motor skill–visuomotor accuracy; (B) gross motor skill; (C) rapid visual information processing; (D) spatial working memory; (E) paired associates learning; and (F) simple reaction time. Figure reproduced from Geertsen et al. (1). Copyright: 2016 Geertsen et al.

detection? Is this the same for all forms of response (i.e. is the lag time the same between the touchscreen and the mouse?) or device (e.g. does your laptop and the laboratory's laptop respond equally quickly?)?

5.2 The effect of hyperthermia and hot ambient conditions on cognitive function

In many sporting events, athletes are required to make complex and challenging decisions e.g. deciding when to alter self-selected pace in a race or deciding when to pass or shoot in a game of football and the athlete requires a high level of cognitive function (ideally in all of the domains) as well as physical prowess to be successful. As covered in the previous chapter, the effect of high ambient temperatures on exercise performance and capacity is well established; however, the effect on cognitive performance is less well known.

It has been proposed that cognitive function may be more sensitive to environmental stress than exercise performance (2), and due to the complex nature of sport, any impairment may compromise sporting performance (e.g. your athlete might be able to continue to run but may not be able to react quick enough to deal with an oncoming opponent) and may also have serious health and safety implications (3). Hot environmental exposure increases subjective feelings of fatigue and discomfort (4;5), and also the frequency of unsafe behaviours (6) whilst elevated body temperatures increase error rate and therefore reduces efficiency and task capability (7).

The effect that hyperthermia has on cognitive function is a complex one with many intertwined variables but it has been suggested that there are four main research variables, or factors, that researchers must consider when investigating the effect of high ambient temperatures on psychological and cognitive performance (8):

1. Environment e.g. air temperature, radiant temperature, air velocity, humidity, clothing
2. Person e.g. training status, skill level, personality, motivation, experience
3. Task e.g. sensory, perceptual, cognitive, team versus individual, open skill versus closed skill
4. Situation e.g. training, competition, crowd presence versus no crowd, high-stakes versus low-stakes, timing

Each of these factors (and their subfactors) interacts to dictate an outcome response (or behaviour) and because this response is a function of these four factors it is unsurprising that the effects of thermal stress and strain on cognitive function are variable and situation specific.

Quick question: If we assume that the environmental ("Environment") stress is the same, which of the following would you expect to have a greater impairment in cognitive function?

* *A well-trained, experienced, and highly motivated athlete in competition*
* *An untrained, inexperienced athlete lacking in motivation in competition*

It is important to understand the effects of passive and active heat stress across a range of domains of cognition, because each of the components of cognition will interact to affect behaviour, and overall sporting performance (9). Due to the many combinations of these four factors (and subfactors), there are many different research designs that have been used to research some, or all, components of cognitive function and the many methodological differences (e.g. a lack of consistency across studies in terms of heating strategies and cognitive tasks used) have resulted in equivocal data. Although there is no definitive answer regarding the magnitude of the effect that hyperthermia has on cognitive function, it is well accepted that cognitive function is impaired by severe hyperthermia (8) and it appears that cognitive disturbances occur once there is an increase in core body temperature above a threshold temperature (10). The magnitude and direction of the effect are dependent upon the complexity of the task (11), and while short-duration, simple cognitive tests appear unaffected (12), hyperthermia appears to impair complex alternatives (13;14). Many complex, cognitive tasks are undertaken by athletes and so any decrease in cognitive function coupled with increases in error rate, perception of fatigue, and unsafe choice selection frequency could have catastrophic consequences for an athlete. A good example here is Formula One motor racing. Formula One drivers are required to navigate a complex track while competing with other drivers in conditions that can exceed 25°C (WBGT; Singapore Grand Prix) at speeds of ~200 k·h^{-1} while sometimes only centimetres from a crash barrier, opponent's car, or wall. Maintaining cognitive function is obviously very important in this situation, as any small error (e.g. slight turn of the wheel or momentary lack of concentration) could result in a high-speed crash!

5.2.1 Passive hyperthermia

Passive hyperthermia models provide researchers with the opportunity to look at the effects that increase body temperature on cognitive function without all of the confounding effects of exercise. While passive hyperthermia will change physiological variables other than just core body temperature (e.g. heart rate will also increase), the magnitude of these other disturbances is likely to be lower than if exercise is used. Unfortunately, there is little consensus in the literature at present regarding the effect that passive heating has on cognitive function largely due to differences in study design. As mentioned, there are a number of ways in which cognitive function and hyperthermia studies can differ, and specifically these include:

- Different magnitudes of increase in core body temperature
- Different magnitudes of increase in skin temperature
- Different levels of thermal comfort and sensation (which is closely related to skin temperature)
- Different methods of heating
- Differences in the complexity of the cognitive function test
- Differences in the domain of the cognitive task e.g. is it assessing

It appears that a moderate elevation in core body temperature (~38°C) improves simple and complex reaction time, attention, executive function, and vigilance cognitive tasks (15–17) but the benefit may be lost once core body temperature is further elevated above a threshold range of 38.2–38.7°C (11;15). Once core body temperature increases above this threshold of ~38.5°C, complex cognitive function is impaired with specific impairments in working memory (18;19), executive function (16), and attention (16–18). Passive heat exposure lengthens response times in perception tasks; however, a trade-off appears to occur whereby accuracy improves (20). The slowing of response times for complex visual perception, alongside an improvement in accuracy, has been reported elsewhere (21) suggesting that resources are reallocated to preserve accuracy at the expense of time but this is not always observed (11). Response times for simple executive function tasks marginally improve following 1 h of heat exposure, suggesting an increase in conduction velocity, but complex executive function tasks are slower (20). The extent of the impairment appears to depend on the magnitude of hyperthermia and the complexity of the task with the performance of simple tasks unaffected at core body temperatures of ~39°C – the temperature at which complex task performance is consistently impaired (11;22;23). It appears that cognitive tasks that require lower levels of attention and focus are less vulnerable to hyperthermia (23;24) but eventually hyperthermia will negatively impact on tasks of all levels of complexity with even simple tasks impaired when core body temperature reaches ~40°C (15).

5.2.2 Active hyperthermia

To add to the aforementioned complexity of cognitive function and hyperthermia studies, there is a desire and a need to answer ecologically valid research questions. As a result, while investigating the effect that passive hyperthermia has on cognitive function provides valuable information regarding the responses and mechanisms explaining them, in order to be able to apply the data in an exercise setting, it is important to understand the effect that active hyperthermia (i.e. exercise-induced increases in core body temperature) has on cognitive function.

It has been shown that exercise alone can improve cognitive function (25;26) (e.g. there is small positive effect of exercise alone on executive function and information processing (26)) and this improvement has been linked to an increase in arousal. Exercise can improve cognitive performance on tasks performed both during and following exercise (26) although the benefit seems small and depends on a number of factors. The benefit seems greatest for fit individuals who perform exercise for at least 20 min, and while any intensity offers a benefit to cognitive function during exercise, lower intensity exercise appears beneficial for cognitive performance assessed once the bout has ended (26). Post-exercise cognitive function may be impaired if the exercise intensity is too high and results in the onset of fatigue – something which can reduce choice reaction task performance (27). Increased arousal might counteract the decrease observed in mental performance with fatigue, especially when task demand is low (28) but the increase in arousal does not compensate for the fatigue-related impairments during complex tasks.

Once you add heat in to the equation not only do you have a complex relationship between exercise, arousal, fatigue, and cognitive function, you also add other confounding variables related to the increased physiological and perceptual strain. For example, increased core body temperatures result in increases in sweat loss and sweat rate which can lead to a hypohydrated state (see Chapters 2 and 8). Hypohydration has been linked to impaired cognitive function (29) but it does not always impair such performance (30). Smith et al. (29) reported that golf-specific skill performance was impaired when experienced golfers (~3 handicap) were ~1% hypohydrated by 12 h of fluid restriction but recently a study in which elite female field hockey players were dehydrated by passive hyperthermia it was reported that cognitive function was unaffected by ~2% body mass losses following intermittent exercise (30). Response times during executive function, complex visuomotor and serial working memory tasks were improved by exposure to hot environmental conditions, and intermittent exercise improved response time regardless of the environmental conditions or hydration status of the participant (30). It seems likely that elite athletes are better at preserving cognitive function when hypohydrated probably because they are more accustomed to having to perform in a hypohydrated state (30) but also that fluid restriction may cause other effects (e.g. impaired participant comfort) that impair cognitive function. The majority of studies that report a decline in cognitive performance following dehydration do so after adopting such an approach.

The topic of active hyperthermia and its effects on cognitive function have also been investigated in occupational settings. In one such investigation that closely mimicked the demands of military service, participants undertook 2.5 h of low-intensity (2–4 $km·h^{-1}$) marching performed in hot ambient conditions (36°C; 60% relative humidity) whilst wearing full combat gear and body armour. There was no effect on cognitive functioning (vigilance, three-term reasoning, filtering, verbal working memory, divided attention, and perceptual reaction time) despite elevations in body temperature (+1.5°C) and cardiovascular strain (4). As discussed, exercise can offset some of the impairment often observed in cognitive function but it is also possible that in a more stressful and/or physiologically demanding situation, cognitive function might have been impaired because the 2.5 h march was shorter than the 4–8 h that military personnel would be expected to march for.

Despite the range of data, it seems likely that active hyperthermia offers a benefit to cognitive function until physiological strain exceeds a benefit threshold. The benefit is likely to come from the initial moderate increase in core body temperature and the added benefit of the exercise itself but there will come a point where the physiological and perceptual strain is too great and hyperthermia, discomfort, and/or fatigue will impair cognitive function. This threshold is likely to depend on a number of factors, such as task complexity, the extent of physiological strain, the athlete's familiarity with the task and level of strain, and the intensity of the exercise and so will differ between athletes.

5.3 Theories of why cognitive function is influenced by hyperthermia

As discussed, the effect that heat stress and strain has on cognitive function is a complex one – small increases in core body temperature can improve cognitive function, but once physiological strain is severe, complex cognitive tasks are impaired. The exact mechanisms for the initial improvement and then impairment are likely to be multifaceted and intertwined and technological advances in measuring and observing responses within the brain (e.g. functional magnetic resonance imaging (fMRI) and electroencephalography (EEG)) may help establish the mechanism(s) over the coming years.

This section will help you to address Problem 5.1: "How can you minimising the effect of exercise in the heat on the cognitive function of your athlete?" because it discusses what might explain the impairment.

You are the coach of an elite field hockey player who is an integral member of the team but whose decision-making declines markedly when the level of thermal stress is high. Field hockey allows for rolling substitutions and so it is typical for players to routinely spend a few minutes off the pitch between bouts of high-intensity exercise. What intervention(s) could you try in order to minimise the impairment in decision-making that was previously observed?

5.3.1 Why is cognitive function improved by moderate increases in core body temperature?

The reasons for the improved cognitive function following small increases in core body temperature are unknown but increases in arousal (31) and decreases in thermal comfort have been implicated (32). Increased arousal has been linked to improvements in cognitive function in cooler conditions and it is possible that this is due to the small increases in core body temperature that are observed during exercise in cooler conditions. The increase in arousal may have a neurotransmitter basis (31). As discussed in Chapter 5, exercise performance in hot conditions may be mediated by dopamine concentrations and similar hypotheses have been made regarding cognitive performance – namely that small increases in core body temperature may elevate dopamine concentrations and improve cognitive function (33). It has also been proposed that a small increase in core body temperature may decrease thermal comfort resulting in athletes deliberately investing a greater amount of cognitive effort into a task to compensate for the increased perception of discomfort (32).

5.3.2 Why is cognitive function impaired by severe increases in core body temperature?

Impaired cognitive performance at higher core body temperatures may be caused by a reduction in cortical activity (34;35) and an inhibition of output intensity from the prefrontal cortex (36;37). Brainwaves (or oscillations) can be divided into five distinct bands (delta, theta, alpha, beta, and gamma) based upon their frequency and each frequency band is associated with different states of brain functioning. In the field of exercise, thermoregulation, and cognitive function, low-frequency theta (frequency of 3–8 Hz) and alpha waves (frequency of 8–13 Hz), and high-frequency beta waves (frequency of 13–30 Hz) have received the most attention. Decreased beta wave activity is linked to higher ratings of perceived exertion (38) and an increase in the ratio of low-to-high frequency brainwaves (an indicator or reduced arousal) is observed during sleep, hyperthermic exercise (38), and when brain temperature is high (39). It has been proposed that cognitive performance may be impaired when hot because there is a greater requirement for neuronal resources when experiencing thermal strain. As core temperature increases, there is an increase in the amplitude and a decrease in the latency of steady-state visually evoked potentials (a measure of brain electrical activity) in the frontal lobe (involved in working memory tasks) and in the occipital and parietal regions (involved in vigilance tasks) (40;41). This increase in neural resources usage persists until they become overloaded (40), suggesting that there is a limit to cognitive capacity (42). Hyperthermia appears to be an additional stress that can contribute to an overloading of the resources and interferes with complex cognitive processes (11). The impairment in cognitive function overserved when core body temperature is high does not appear to be related to reductions in cerebral blood flow or substrate delivery (43;44) but may be linked to cortisol concentrations (45). There is a relationship between cortisol concentrations and working memory task performance (45) and it has been hypothesised that cortisol may trigger the reallocation of resources from the frontal region of the brain to the emotional centres. fMRI data suggest that hyperthermia increases activation in the temporal lobe during a visual perception task, but decreases activity in the frontal lobe, parietal lobe, and occipital lobe (24) (Figure 5.2). These findings suggest that during passive hyperthermia, the brain can redistribute resources to try and maintain performance in the required domain.

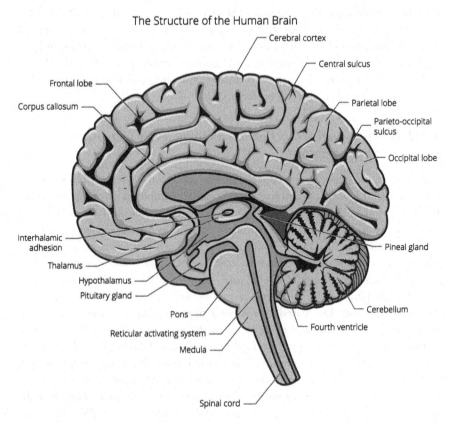

The Structure of the Human Brain

FIGURE 5.2 The human brain.

Simple cognitive tasks are relatively unaffected by hyperthermia and very high core body temperatures appear to be required to impair such performance. In contrast, for complex cognitive tasks, there appears to be an inverted u-shape relationship between core body temperature and cognitive function with an initial improvement observed until a core body temperature threshold of ~38.5°C is surpassed after which cognitive performance is impaired. Put another way, complex cognitive tasks generally demonstrate greater vulnerability to the effects of heat, possibly due to draining of neural resources (46), whilst simple task performance can be maintained and this pattern of response aligns nicely with the maximal availability model proposed by Hancock and Warm (46) (Figure 5.3). The maximal availability model suggests that heat competes for, and eventually drains, attentional resources, which explains why a moderate increase in core body temperature improves cognitive function (through the adoption of strategies such as increased attentional focus) but as the level of thermal strain increases, attentional resources are depleted and cognitive function is impaired.

Gaoua et al. (23) sought to test whether cognitive function did decline when under heat stress due to a depletion of resources and used EEG to do so. As mentioned earlier, most EEG studies have looked at the difference between high-frequency (beta waves) and low-frequency (theta and alpha waves) wave lengths. Alpha activity is linked to impaired cognitive processing (48) and

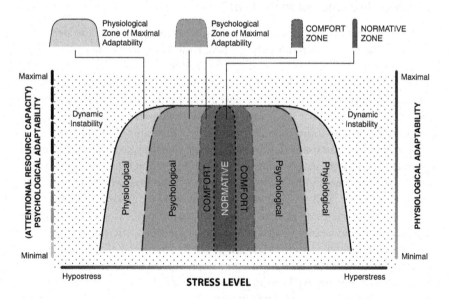

FIGURE 5.3 The maximal adaptability model. Figure reproduced from Roberts et al. (47). Roberts AC, Christopoulos GI, Car J, Soh C, Lu M. Psychobiological factors associated with underground spaces: What can the new era of cognitive neuroscience offer to their study? *Tunnelling and Underground Space Technology* 2016;55:118–34, Copyright (2016) with permission from Elsevier.

decreases during complex tasks (49), whereas theta power over the frontal lobe increases during working memory and concentration tasks (50). The increase in theta wave activity suggests that there is an increase in demand on working memory (51) and it has been proposed that theta oscillations may be the best indicator of mental workload and cognitive fatigue (52). Gaoua et al. (23) observed that the accuracy of responses was reduced in hyperthermic individuals (gastrointestinal temperature = ~39°C) and this was observed alongside an elevation in EEG theta power prior to the commencement of the task. The elevation in theta wave power prior to undertaking a cognitive task suggests that the hyperthermia alone imposed a cognitive load. The authors postulated that this was due to decreases in thermal comfort. During a simple task, theta power was elevated in the hyperthermia trial compared to normothermia, whereas in a more complex test the elevation was similar between each group – these data suggest that during a simpler task, working memory resources are increased to maintain cognitive task performance. The data from Gaoua et al. (23) offer support for the maximal adaptability theory by demonstrating that hyperthermia and cognitive tasks both impose a cognitive load, and when the load is too great (complex tasks), there is an inability to allocate additional resources and so performance declines.

5.3.3 Is it only core temperature changes that can alter cognitive function in the heat?

As discussed in Chapter 2, there are a number of physiological and perceptual responses that occur as a result of heat stress. Responses such as increases in heart rate and sweat rate can alter thermal comfort and sensation and such disturbances may also contribute to the decrements in cognitive function observed – either in tandem with, or irrespective of, the core body temperature change (11;53). We know that how and what an athlete feels when exposed to high ambient temperatures depend on more than just core body temperature (see Chapter 3) and so, unsurprisingly, increases in skin temperature that leads to negative perceptual responses can also negatively influence cognitive function (11;53). Complex cognitive tasks are impaired following passive heat exposure, which increases skin temperature (by ~ 3°C) without elevating core body temperature (54) and with only very small increases in core body temperature (increases of ~0.2°C from baseline) (20) demonstrating that impairments are not solely due to large core body temperature elevations. Malcolm et al. (20) reported that 1 h of passive hyperthermia slowed response times but improved accuracy on the simple and complex tasks. The passive heating elevated skin temperature, core temperature, heart rate, thermal sensation, and felt arousal while reducing the perceived rating of pleasure highlighting that despite the literature, core body temperature is not the only regulator of cognitive performance (20). Skin temperature has a role to play as demonstrated by the fact that cooling the head can preserve some complex cognitive functions (11) and cognitive performance can be impaired in hot conditions when core body temperature is unaffected but skin temperature is elevated (55). Gaoua et al. (54) observed that exposing participants to very hot (50°C; 30 relative humidity) for ~30 min to elevate skin temperature (+ 2.8°C) without increasing core body temperature had no effect on reaction time, latency, or accuracy in simple or complex reaction time tests. It also had no effect on a simple test of executive function but altered complex cognitive task performance. Executive function was impaired with high skin temperatures compared to control – participants responded quicker but due to making errors they took longer to find the correct response (54). Increase in skin temperature that reduces perceived thermal comfort and pleasure has the potential to distract athletes and research participants from cognitive tasks, subsequently impairing performance.

Problem 5.1 revisited. How can you minimise the effect of exercise in the heat on the cognitive function of your athlete?

You are the coach of an elite field hockey player who is an integral member of the team but whose decision-making declines markedly when the level of thermal stress is high. Field hockey allows for rolling substitutions and so it is typical for players to routinely spend a few minutes off the pitch between bouts of high-intensity exercise. What intervention(s) could you try in order to minimise the impairment in decision-making that was previously observed? In order to answer this problem, you will need to consider what might explain the impairment.

Your athlete may experience an initial increase in cognitive function (i.e. decision-making) during the match in hot conditions; however, once their core body temperature (or possibly their perception of core body temperature/thermal strain) exceeds a threshold, the impairment will start to become noticeable. The best way to try and minimise this impairment is to identify the potential reasons for the impairment.

Quick question: Based on the information in Section 5.3, how many possible reasons can you identify?

I think that there are three main reasons that are all related to the magnitude of perceived and/or actual physiological strain experienced.

1. Alterations in thermal comfort

    Decreased thermal comfort has been proposed as one reason to explain the initial improvement in cognitive function observed as core body temperatures increase, as it is thought that athletes may deliberately invest a greater amount of cognitive effort into a task to compensate for the increased perception of discomfort.

2. Alterations in cerebral dopamine concentrations

    Elevations in cerebral concentrations of dopamine have been implicated in the initial improvement in cognitive function; however, it seems likely that, as with exercise performance in the heat (see Chapter 4), cognitive function would become impaired as core body temperature continues to increase and cerebral dopamine concentrations fall.

3. Alterations in brainwave activity

There may be a shift from high-frequency to low-frequency brainwave activity during exercise in the heat and that cognitive function may be impaired due a greater requirement for neuronal resources when experiencing thermal strain. The maximal availability model suggests that heat competes for, and eventually drains, attentional resources which explains why a moderate increase in core body temperature improves cognitive function (through the adoption of strategies such as increased attentional focus) but as the level of thermal strain increases, attentional resources are depleted and cognitive function is impaired.

As mentioned, all three of these potential explanations are heavily related to the actual or perceived physiological strain and so the most likely way to minimise the impairment would be to reduce this.

The demands of the game are very high due to the intermittent nature and so the development of high levels of physiological strain is inevitable; however, you could adopt strategies to minimise the strain before or during the game. For example, you could reduce the initial core body temperature of your athlete by getting them to undertake a structured heat acclimation (see Chapter 6) or pre-cooling intervention (see Chapter 7), or attempt to minimise increases in core body temperature by increasing the frequency of substitutions thereby increasing the ratio of rest to work. The latter of option might not be realistic due to the impact it will have on tactics and match play. Minimising core body temperature increases is likely to be challenging, but fortunately, it is not just core body temperature increases that can impair cognitive function. Increases in skin temperature can also impair cognitive function and appear to do so by decreasing the perceived level of thermal comfort. This suggests that if skin temperature can be lowered and perceived thermal comfort can be increased, then reductions in cognitive function may be able to be attenuated. Localised skin cooling can lower skin temperature and improve thermal comfort and has also been shown to improve cognitive function compared to no cooling. As a result, any intervention that can achieve this alteration in skin temperature and thermal comfort should be adopted e.g. fans, ice vests (see Chapter 7).

If decreased cerebral concentrations of dopamine do play a role in the decreased cognitive function, then any intervention that increases these concentrations should slow or reverse the decline. As mentioned in Chapter 4, there are pharmacological interventions that can do this; however, these are prohibited substances and so can only be recommended to your athlete by a medical doctor.

5.4 Summary

There is a complex range of factors that have the potential to influence cognitive function during hyperthermia and there is still much to establish in this field. The main reasons for the lack of consensus are the differences between studies and the complex, integrated nature of cognitive function (it is an umbrella term with a number of components each of which may respond differently to the same stress or strain). The effect of heat stress and strain on cognitive function appears to be dependent upon the task complexity, the expertise and experience of the athlete, and magnitude of thermal stress and strain experienced. Small increases in actual or perceived thermal strain may improve cognitive function due to increased arousal and/or cognitive effort as a result of increased thermal discomfort but once core body temperatures exceed ~38.5°C, complex cognitive performance is impaired. Simple tasks are less vulnerable to heat stress and strain than more complex ones, and are only impaired by very hot (~40°C) core body temperatures. While elevations in core body temperature appear to benefit and then impair cognitive function, impairments can also be observed without meaningful increases in core body temperature if skin temperatures are increased and perceived levels of thermal comfort and pleasure decrease.

5.5 Self-check quiz

At the start of the chapter you were told that you should know the following by the end of the chapter:

- What is cognitive function and what are its subcomponents?
- How is cognitive function assessed?
- How is cognitive function affected by hyperthermia?
- Why is cognitive function affected by hyperthermia?
- What other factors can affect the cognitive function of athletes competing in hot conditions?

The following self-check quiz will help you see whether the learning outcomes of this chapter have been achieved. Section 5.1 will help you with questions 1–3, the answers to questions 4 and 5 can be found in Section 5.2, and the answers to the others can be found in Section 5.3.

5.5.1 Self-check quiz questions

1. What is cognitive function?
2. What are the five main areas of cognitive function?
3. Are complex or simple tasks more likely to be impaired when an athlete is hot?
4. Above what core body temperature threshold does complex cognitive function appear to deteriorate?
5. Above what core body temperature are simple cognitive tasks impaired?
6. What are the two main reasons used to explain the initial improvement in cognitive function as core body temperature increases?

7. Are decreases in high-frequency (beta) or low-frequency (theta and alpha) brainwave activity linked to decreased arousal and increased ratings of perceived exertion?
8. What model has been proposed by Hancock and Warm to try and explain the impairment in cognitive function observed in the heat?
9. Can cognitive function be impaired if core body temperatures are not high?
10. Why might elevated skin temperature impair cognitive function?

5.5.2 Self-check quiz answers

1. Cognitive function is a measure of the accuracy and efficiency of cortical and subcortical processes in detecting, identifying, and responding to external stimuli i.e. how well can you identify and accurately respond to a stimulus.
2. Executive function, memory, attention, psychomotor speed, and social and emotion cognition.
3. Complex tasks are more vulnerable to high levels of thermal stress and strain.
4. Approximately 38.5°C although impairments have been observed once core body temperature exceeds 38.0–38.2°C.
5. ~40°C.
6. An increase in arousal and a decrease in thermal comfort that causes the athlete to deliberately make more of a cognitive effort into the task to compensate for the increased perception of discomfort.
7. High frequency. Decreased beta wave activity is linked to higher ratings of perceived exertion.
8. The maximal availability model which suggests that heat competes for, and eventually drains, attentional resources.
9. Yes. Impairments have been observed in athletes without elevated core body temperatures.
10. Increase in skin temperature that reduces perceived thermal comfort and pleasure has the potential to distract athletes and research participants from cognitive tasks, subsequently impairing cognitive performance.

References

1 Geertsen SS, Thomas R, Larsen MN, Dahn IM, Andersen JN, Krause-Jensen M, et al. Motor skills and exercise capacity are associated with objective measures of cognitive functions and academic performance in preadolescent children. *PLoS One* 2016;11(8):e0161960.
2 Hancock PA, Vasmatzidis I. Effects of heat stress on cognitive performance: the current state of knowledge. *Int J Hyperthermia* 2003 May;19(3):355–72.
3 Cheung SS. Neuropsychological determinants of exercise tolerance in the heat. *Prog Brain Res* 2007;162:45–60.
4 Caldwell JN, Engelen L, van der Henst C, Patterson MJ, Taylor NA. The interaction of body armor, low-intensity exercise, and hot-humid conditions on physiological strain and cognitive function. *Mil Med* 2011 May;176(5):488–93.
5 Tyler CJ, Sunderland C. The effect of ambient temperature on the reliability of a preloaded treadmill time-trial. *Int J Sports Med* 2008 May 6;29:812–6.

6 Ramsey JD, Burford CL, Beshir MY, Jensen RC. Effects of workplace thermal conditions on safe work behaviour. *J Safety Res* 1983;14:105–14.

7 Allan JR, Gibson TM. Separation of the effects of raised skin and core temperature on performance of a pursuit rotor task. *Aviat Space Environ Med* 1979 Jul;50(7):678–82.

8 Johnson RF, Kobrick JL. Psychological aspects of military performance in hot environments. In: Pandolf KB, Burr RE, editors. Medical aspects of harsh environments, Volume 1. Washington, DC: Borden Institute; 2001. p. 135–59.

9 Allard F, Burnett N. Skill in sport. *Can J Exp Psych* 1985;39(2):294–312.

10 Faerevik H, Reinertsen RE. Effects of wearing aircrew protective clothing on physiological and cognitive responses under various ambient conditions. *Ergonomics* 2003 Jun 20;46(8):780–99.

11 Gaoua N, Racinais S, Grantham J, El MF. Alterations in cognitive performance during passive hyperthermia are task dependent. *Int J Hyperthermia* 2011;27(1):1–9.

12 Amos D, Hansen R, Lau WM, Michalski JT. Physiological and cognitive performance of soldiers conducting routine patrol and reconnaissance operations in the tropics. *Mil Med* 2000 Dec;165(12):961–6.

13 Cian C, Barraud PA, Melin B, Raphel C. Effects of fluid ingestion on cognitive function after heat stress or exercise-induced dehydration. *Int J Psychophysiol* 2001 Nov;42(3):243–51.

14 Fine BJ, Kobrick JL. Effect of heat and chemical protective clothing on cognitive performance. Natick: USARIEM; 1985. Report No.: M4/86.

15 Bandelow S, Maughan R, Shirreffs S, Ozgunen K, Kurdak S, Ersoz G, et al. The effects of exercise, heat, cooling and rehydration strategies on cognitive function in football players. *Scand J Med Sci Sports* 2010 Oct;20 Suppl 3:148–60.

16 Schlader ZJ, Gagnon D, Adams A, Rivas E, Cullum CM, Crandall CG. Cognitive and perceptual responses during passive heat stress in younger and older adults. *Am J Physiol Regul Integr Comp Physiol* 2015 May 15;308(10):R847–R854.

17 Simmons SE, Saxby BK, McGlone FP, Jones DA. The effect of passive heating and head cooling on perception, cardiovascular function and cognitive performance in the heat. *Eur J Appl Physiol* 2008 Sep;104(2):271–80.

18 Lieberman HR, Bathalon GP, Falco CM, Kramer FM, Morgan CA, III, Niro P. Severe decrements in cognition function and mood induced by sleep loss, heat, dehydration, and undernutrition during simulated combat. *Biol Psychiatry* 2005 Feb 15;57(4):422–9.

19 Morley J, Beauchamp G, Suyama J, Guyette FX, Reis SE, Callaway CW, et al. Cognitive function following treadmill exercise in thermal protective clothing. *Eur J Appl Physiol* 2012 May;112(5):1733–40.

20 Malcolm RA, Cooper S, Folland JP, Tyler CJ, Sunderland C. Passive heat exposure alters perception and executive function. *Front Physiol* 2018;9:585.

21 Hancock PA, Dirkin GR. Central and peripheral visual choice-reaction time under conditions of induced cortical hyperthermia. *Percept Mot Skills* 1982 Apr;54(2):395–402.

22 Racinais S, Gaoua N, Grantham J. Hyperthermia impairs short-term memory and peripheral motor drive transmission. *J Physiol* 2008 Oct 1;586(19):4751–62.

23 Gaoua N, Herrera CP, Periard JD, El MF, Racinais S. Effect of passive hyperthermia on working memory resources during simple and complex cognitive tasks. *Front Psychol* 2017;8:2290.

24 Liu K, Sun G, Li B, Jiang Q, Yang X, Li M, et al. The impact of passive hyperthermia on human attention networks: an fMRI study. *Behav Brain Res* 2013 Apr 15;243:220–30.

25 Adam GE, Carter R, III, Cheuvront SN, Merullo DJ, Castellani JW, Lieberman HR, et al. Hydration effects on cognitive performance during military tasks in temperate and cold environments. *Physiol Behav* 2008 Mar 18;93(4–5):748–56.

26 Chang YK, Labban JD, Gapin JI, Etnier JL. The effects of acute exercise on cognitive performance: a meta-analysis. *Brain Res* 2012 May 9;1453:87–101.

27 Lorist MM, Kernell D, Meijman TF, Zijdewind I. Motor fatigue and cognitive task performance in humans. *J Physiol* 2002 Nov 15;545(Pt 1):313–9.

28 Razmjou S. Mental workload in heat: toward a framework for analyses of stress states. *Aviat Space Environ Med* 1996 Jun;67(6):530–8.

29 Smith MF, Newell AJ, Baker MR. Effect of acute mild dehydration on cognitive-motor performance in golf. *J Strength Cond Res* 2012 Nov;26(11):3075–80.

30 Macleod H, Cooper S, Bandelow S, Malcolm R, Sunderland C. Effects of heat stress and dehydration on cognitive function in elite female field hockey players. *BMC Sports Sci Med Rehabil* 2018;10:12.

31 McMorris T, Swain J, Smith M, Corbett J, Delves S, Sale C, et al. Heat stress, plasma concentrations of adrenaline, noradrenaline, 5-hydroxytryptamine and cortisol, mood state and cognitive performance. *Int J Psychophysiol* 2006 Aug;61(2):204–15.

32 Flouris AD, Schlader ZJ. Human behavioral thermoregulation during exercise in the heat. *Scand J Med Sci Sports* 2015 Jun;25 Suppl 1:52–64.

33 Robbins TW, Everitt BJ. A role for mesencephalic dopamine in activation: commentary on Berridge (2006). *Psychopharmacology (Berl)* 2007 Apr;191(3):433–7.

34 De PK, Roelands B, Marusic U, Tellez HF, Knaepen K, Meeusen R. Brain mapping after prolonged cycling and during recovery in the heat. *J Appl Physiol (1985)* 2013 Nov 1;115(9):1324–31.

35 Nybo L, Nielsen B. Hyperthermia and central fatigue during prolonged exercise in humans. *J Appl Physiol* 2001 Sep;91(3):1055–60.

36 Olausson H, Charron J, Marchand S, Villemure C, Strigo IA, Bushnell MC. Feelings of warmth correlate with neural activity in right anterior insular cortex. *Neurosci Lett* 2005 Nov 25;389(1):1–5.

37 Schmidt L, LeBreton M, Clery-Melin ML, Daunizeau J, Pessiglione M. Neural mechanisms underlying motivation of mental versus physical effort. *PLoS Biol* 2012 Feb;10(2):e1001266.

38 Nielsen B, Hyldig T, Bidstrup F, Gonzalez-Alonso J, Christoffersen GR. Brain activity and fatigue during prolonged exercise in the heat. *Pflugers Arch* 2001 Apr;442(1):41–8.

39 Eshel GM, Safar P. The role of the central nervous system in heatstroke: reversible profound depression of cerebral activity in a primate model. *Aviat Space Environ Med* 2002 Apr;73(4):327–32.

40 Hocking C, Silberstein RB, Lau WM, Stough C, Roberts W. Evaluation of cognitive performance in the heat by functional brain imaging and psychometric testing. *Comp Biochem Physiol A Mol Integr Physiol* 2001 Apr;128(4):719–34.

41 Silberstein RB, Schier MA, Pipingas A, Ciorciari J, Wood SR, Simpson DG. Steady-state visually evoked potential topography associated with a visual vigilance task. *Brain Topogr* 1990;3(2):337–47.

42 Baars BJ. How does a serial, integrated and very limited stream of consciousness emerge from a nervous system that is mostly unconscious, distributed, parallel and of enormous capacity? *Ciba Found Symp* 1993;174:282–90.

43 Nybo L, Moller K, Volianitis S, Nielsen B, Secher NH. Effects of hyperthermia on cerebral blood flow and metabolism during prolonged exercise in humans. *J Appl Physiol* 2002 Jul;93(1):58–64.

44 Schlader ZJ, Lucas RA, Pearson J, Crandall CG. Hyperthermia does not alter the increase in cerebral perfusion during cognitive activation. *Exp Physiol* 2013 Nov;98(11):1597–607.

45 Kirschbaum C, Wolf OT, May M, et al. Stress- and treatmentinduced elevations of cortisol levels associated with impaired declarative memory in healthy adults. *Life Sci.* 1996;58:1475–83.

46 Hancock PA, Warm JS. A dynamic model of stress and sustained attention. *Hum Factors* 1989 Oct;31(5):519–37.

47 Roberts AC, Christopoulos GI, Car J, Soh C, Lu M. Psycho-biological factors associated with underground spaces: what can the new era of cognitive neuroscience offer to their study? *Tunnelling and Underground Space Technol* 2016;55:118–34.
48 Lang W, Lang M, Kornhuber A, Diekmann V, Kornhuber HH. Event-related EEG-spectra in a concept formation task. *Hum Neurobiol* 1988;6(4):295–301.
49 Gundel A, Wilson GF. Topographical changes in the ongoing EEG related to the difficulty of mental tasks. *Brain Topogr* 1992;5(1):17–25.
50 Gevins A, Smith ME, McEvoy L, Yu D. High-resolution EEG mapping of cortical activation related to working memory: effects of task difficulty, type of processing, and practice. *Cereb Cortex* 1997 Jun;7(4):374–85.
51 Kahana MJ, Sekuler R, Caplan JB, Kirschen M, Madsen JR. Human theta oscillations exhibit task dependence during virtual maze navigation. *Nature* 1999 Jun 24;399(6738):781–4.
52 Smith ME, Gevins A, Brown H, Karnik A, Du R. Monitoring task loading with multivariate EEG measures during complex forms of human-computer interaction. *Hum Factors* 2001;43(3):366–80.
53 Gaoua N. Cognitive function in hot environments: a question of methodology. *Scand J Med Sci Sports* 2010 Oct;20 Suppl 3:60–70.
54 Gaoua N, Grantham J, Racinais S, El MF. Sensory displeasure reduces complex cognitive performance in the heat. *J Env Psych* 2012;32:158–63.
55 Gaoua N, Grantham J, El MF, Girard O, Racinais S. Cognitive decrements do not follow neuromuscular alterations during passive heat exposure. *Int J Hyperthermia* 2011;27(1):10–9.

6

HEAT ACCLIMATION AND ACCLIMATISATION

What should you know by the end of the chapter?

As discussed in Chapters 4 and 5, exercise and cognitive performance can be impaired by hot environmental conditions and the resulting elevations in physiological and perceptual strain. Strategies to minimise or prevent the impaired performance are highly sought by athletes and coaches and as a result a number of strategies have been proposed and adopted. This chapter will discuss the most potentially effective strategy – heat acclimation/acclimatisation. By the end of this chapter you should know:

- What is the difference between heat acclimation and heat acclimatisation? Do the different approaches have different effects on exercise performance and the physiological responses to exercise in the heat?
- The different heat adaptation protocols used and what their strengths and weaknesses are
- Differences between active and passive heat acclimation
- Physiological, perceptual, and molecular responses to heat acclimation
- Whether heat adaptation can offer a benefit in other environmental extremes
- The rate and extent of heat acclimation decay
- Heat reacclimation and decay considerations

Key terms for this chapter

Adaptation threshold	A physiological threshold that must be exceeded in order for adaptation to occur
HA	Heat acclimation. Artificially induced heat adaptation (e.g. using a laboratory-based environmental chamber)

Heat acclimation decay	The loss of beneficial adaptation to heat due to the removal of a sufficient thermal impulse
Heat acclimatisation	Heat adaptations induced by natural exposure (e.g. warm-weather training camps or domestic exposure to elevated ambient temperatures)
HR	Heat reacclimation. Making beneficial adaptations to heat that have been lost following a period of heat acclimation decay
Isothermic hyperthermia	Exercise and heat stress are manipulated to achieve a target core body temperature (often 38.5°C). Also referred to as controlled hyperthermia
LTHA	Long-term heat acclimation. Heat acclimation regimens involving more than 14 heat exposures
MTHA	Moderate-term heat acclimation. Heat acclimation regimens involving 8–14 heat exposures
STHA	Short-term heat acclimation. Heat acclimation regimens involving seven or less heat exposures
Thermal impulse	An increase in core body temperature which results in heat adaptations

Problem 6.1: Heat acclimation on a budget

You are a volunteer coach for a local Scottish football team that has been invited to take part in a summer tournament in Barcelona. The temperature is forecast to be 30–35°C and you would like to prepare the team for the heat prior to flying out because your first match is scheduled to take place 24 h after you land in Barcelona. You and the team fly out in 14 days so you have ti me to prepare but unfortunately you do not have access to an environmental chamber and the local temperatures are not expected to exceed 20°C. What can you do to prepare your athletes for the heat that is inexpensive and does not require any specialist equipment?

Problem 6.2: Optimising heat acclimation for the elite athlete

You are the head physiologist for the National Athletic Association and planning for an upcoming competition abroad where the temperatures are expected to exceed 30°C. You have been instructed to develop a four-week plan to help the marathon runners deal with the conditions. Your athletes will arrive at the competition one week before it is due to start but fortunately your domestic training facility has an environmental chamber on site. What will you do?

6.1 "Heat acclimation" versus "heat acclimatisation"

Heat acclimation (HA) and heat acclimatisation describe the adaptations made by the body following repeated bouts of heat exposure that reduce the physiological and perceptual strain experienced during subsequent bouts. HA describes artificially induced heat adaptation (e.g. using a laboratory-based environmental chamber), whereas *heat acclimatisation* describes adaptations induced by natural exposure (e.g. warm-weather training camps or domestic exposure to elevated

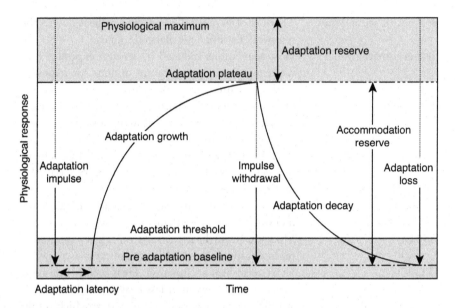

FIGURE 6.1 Characteristics of physiological adaptation highlighting the accommodation reserve range and the effects of exceeding this on adaptation to
heat. Reproduced from Taylor (2) with permission from John Wiley and
Sons. Copyright 2014 American Physiological Society.

ambient temperatures) (1). I always remember the difference because acclimatisation is the longer word, and it takes longer to get somewhere far away (e.g. a
warm-weather camp)!

In order for an athlete to adapt to high ambient temperatures, a HA or acclimatisation programme needs to provide the body with a series of thermal impulses
(elevations in core body temperature) that exceed an adaptation threshold and facilitates adaptation growth within the accommodation reserve range (2) (Figure 6.1).

If the impulses are insufficient, adaptation will either occur suboptimally or
not at all and so the effectiveness of a HA programme depends on the extent to
which body temperature can be elevated and maintained once elevated. Athletes
frequently arrive at the competition venue a number of days in advance if hot
weather is expected in order to acclimatise; however, this is not always possible
and so many athletes undertake HA prior to leaving. HA can be expensive and
this may explain why only ~15% of athletes who responded to a questionnaire
had undertaken HA prior to the 2015 IAAF World Championships in Beijing
despite hot weather being forecast (3).

6.1.1 Does it matter whether you undertake HA or heat acclimatisation?

The answer to this question is currently unknown. Adaptations are made to a
given stressor, and so if the stressor is the same, the adaptations are unlikely to

differ. In the altitude literature, there is currently a debate about whether the responses to hypobaric (low atmospheric pressure) hypoxia differ from those to normobaric (sea-level atmospheric pressure) hypoxia. The responses to hypobaric and normobaric hypoxia may differ for a number of reasons, including differences in air resistance, partial pressure, atmospheric pressure, and oxygen levels although the data are equivocal. When comparing HA versus heat acclimatisation, the stressor is singular – heat – although as discussed in Chapter 3, a number of environmental factors combine to create the heat stress e.g. solar radiation, airflow, humidity.

The responses to acclimation and acclimatisation would probably be identical if the heat stress was exactly the same; however, this is unlikely to ever be the case. Environmental factors such as solar radiation and airflow are often missing or provided at suboptimal levels in HA protocols, whereas athletes undertaking heat acclimatisation would find it more difficult to avoid elevated temperatures. Most HA protocols take place in an environmental chamber or heated room and so as soon as the athlete leaves the room the thermal stress is removed whereas an athlete would need to seek an air-conditioned space (e.g. hotel room) to escape the heat when undertaking heat acclimatisation. For this reason, the adaptations to heat acclimatisation may be greater as a result because of greater heat exposure – data to support this will be discussed later in the chapter.

Because it is unknown whether the responses differ between HA and acclimatisation, HA will be used as a collective term to describe HA and heat acclimatisation unless explicitly stated otherwise in this chapter.

6.2 Different HA methods

The *average* HA protocol involves nine consecutive HA sessions, each lasting 105 min of exercise in hot conditions (40°C, 40% relative humidity) (4) but the actual protocols used vary considerably. Despite the interest in HA both in the research world and in the sporting one, there is little consensus on what makes for an optimal programme and this is largely due to the number of ways in which a programme could differ – namely the frequency, duration, intensity, or type (summarised in Table 6.1).

This section contains a lot of information and will help you answer both of the problems posed at the start of the chapter:

Problem 6.1: Heat acclimation on a budget: You are a volunteer coach for a local Scottish football team that has been invited to take part in a summer tournament in Barcelona. The temperature is forecast to be 30–35°C and you would like to prepare the team for the heat prior to flying out because your first match is scheduled to take place 24 h after you land in Barcelona. You and the team fly out in 14 days so you have time to prepare but unfortunately you do not have access to an environmental chamber and the local temperatures are not expected to exceed 20°C. What can you do to prepare your athletes for the heat that is inexpensive and does not require any specialist equipment?

Problem 6.2: Optimising heat acclimation for the elite athlete: You are the head physiologist for the National Athletic Association and planning for an upcoming competition abroad where the temperatures are expected to exceed 30°C. You have been instructed to develop a four-week plan to help the marathon runners deal with the conditions. Your athletes will arrive at the competition one week before it is due to start but fortunately your domestic training facility has an environmental chamber on site. What will you do?

6.2.1 Frequency

The frequency of HA sessions used in elite sport and researched in the laboratories around the world can differ markedly, often because individuals are striving to balance the demands of pre-competition preparation with those of heat adaptation. Prior to competition, athletes are often attempting to taper while trying to overcome the disturbances in routine that accompany a competition and if they also want to adapt to high ambient temperatures often they are looking for as a quick an adaptation period as possible – even if this results in suboptimal adaptation. In order to help standardise HA terminology, the following descriptors have been proposed for describing the frequency of HA:

- Short-term heat acclimation (STHA): <7 exposures
- Moderate-term heat acclimation (MTHA): 8–14 exposures
- Long-term heat acclimation (LTHA): >15 exposures)

These exposures can be experienced on consecutive or non-consecutive days; however, little data exist investigating the effect of this. Most HA studies involve consecutive days of heat exposure and such an approach may be more efficient at inducing adaptation to heat. Ten consecutive days has a similar effect to ten days undertaken over a three-week period, so if time is an issue, consecutive days should be used, but if it is less of an issue, adaptation can still occur if HA sessions take place every 2–3 days (5).

6.2.2 Duration

The beneficial effect of HA on performance is dependent on the duration of heat exposure with longer durations resulting in greater performance benefits (4). There is little consensus on the optimal duration of each HA session with daily bouts lasting 60 min (6) and 100 min (7) proposed. Longer but less thermally demanding HA sessions (e.g. lower ambient conditions and/or lower endogenous heat production) are likely to offer less of a thermal impulse, and therefore a lower adaptation stimulus, than shorter more thermally challenging HA sessions. The HA sessions investigated to date have used session durations ranging from 27 to 300 min (mean duration 105 ± 62 min) (4).

6.2.3 Intensity

The magnitude of adaptation is also dependent upon the intensity of the heat stress and strain. Improvements in exercise performance and beneficial adaptations in sweat response and plasma volume change following HA are moderately linked to the temperature used for HA; however, the temperatures used are rather homogenous. The temperature and humidity used range from 25°C to 55°C and 13% to 100%, respectively, with a mean thermal stress of 40°C and 40% relative humidity (4) (estimated wet-bulb globe temperature = 38°C; see Chapter 3 for more information related to wet-bulb globe temperature). The use of an ambient temperature in excess of natural heat exposure is required for heat adaptation and this should be considered when acclimating individuals who reside in warm conditions and have a high level of natural heat acclimatisation. Heat stress intensity should be progressively increased during the HA regimen until individuals are adapting to the desired temperatures in order to maintain a balance between heat adaptation and training adaptation.

Most HA studies use prolonged, sub-maximal exercise; however, greater endogenous heat strain can be created by increasing the exercise intensity. Little data exist directly comparing difference intensities, but adaptations caused by 30–35 min of moderate-intensity exercise (75% maximal oxygen consumption) are similar to those induced by 60 min of lower intensity exercise (50% maximal oxygen consumption) (8). If exercise intensity is being adjusted to provide a sufficient adaptation impulse, it is crucial that absolute intensity is increased with adaptation, otherwise the relative intensity will drop, and the magnitude of heat adaptation will be compromised (2). If time is limited, increasing the exercise intensity may facilitate heat adaptation more efficiently; however, although high-intensity interval STHA can reduce ratings of perceived exertion (often abbreviated to RPE) and thermal comfort (9), improve maximal sprint performance, and lower both core body temperature and heart rate (10), longer duration performance (20 km time trial) has been shown to be either unchanged (10) or impaired (11). This suggests that exercise specificity should be considered when designing HA regimens. High-intensity exercise in the heat may disrupt the normal hypothalamic–pituitary–adrenal axis stress response (12) by overly taxing the body by the dual stressors of heat and exercise. This could have a negative impact on recovery and performance.

6.2.4 Type

The HA phenotype is generally achieved using one of three HA regimen types:

1. Self-regulated/self-paced work HA
2. Constant work HA
3. Isothermic/controlled hyperthermia HA

6.2.4.1 Self-regulated/self-paced work HA

The self-regulated work model requires individuals to self-select their exercise intensity based upon their own perceived levels of discomfort caused by the heat exposure or other available cues. For example, you may ask an athlete to maintain a "steady jog" or exercise at a "15" on the 6–20 rating of perceived exertion scale and, depending on how they feel, the intensity self-selected will differ. Allowing individuals to self-select the exercise intensity means that it can be difficult (sometimes impossible) to quantify the thermal strain experienced thereby ensuring that the progressive overload required for adaptation to occur is problematic (2). Having said this, self-regulated HA protocols may be more effective than the other approaches at enhancing exercise performance if well-motivated participants are involved because they appear to self-select an exercise intensity sufficient to result in adaptations (4).

6.2.4.2 Constant work HA

The constant work model is, as the name suggests, one that involves the athlete(s) working at a set intensity throughout the HA programme. It is the most commonly used method, especially in military settings, because it is easy to simultaneously acclimate multiple individuals (4). This model has been used extensively; however, recent studies have moved away from this approach because at a given intensity different individuals will have different relative thermal loads. As a result, this model does not lend itself to a uniform magnitude of adaptation between individuals, e.g. a fitter athlete working at the same absolute intensity (e.g. 165 W) as a less fit athlete will be exercising at a lower relative intensity and as a result will be under less physiological (thermal) strain.

6.2.4.3 Isothermic/controlled hyperthermia HA

A relatively new HA approach is the controlled hyperthermia one which has been designed to overcome the issues associated with the need for a progressive and measurable overload. Repeated bouts of identical thermal stress will not induce optimal heat adaptation because, as adaptation occurs, the magnitude of physiological strain will be reduced. The work undertaken in the controlled hyperthermia model is increased as adaptation occurs to maintain the thermal impulse required for adaptation. The controlled hyperthermia model can be active or passive and is also referred to as the "isothermal model" because a target core body temperature (often 38.5°C) is often sought in this approach. As resting core body temperature lowers with adaptation, a greater rise is required to reach this target and so more work is required to be performed – this maintains the thermal impulse. Due to the difficulty in measuring core body temperature in elite settings, recently there has been some attention on using heart rate, rather than core body temperature, to set the intensity because as adaptation occurs, heart rate reduces and so by increasing the exercise intensity to maintain a predetermined heart rate, continued heat adaptation should be possible (13).

6.2.4.4 Active versus passive HA

Passive HA can occur naturally (e.g. athletes training in warm gymnasiums or workers working in a warm office) or can be artificially induced in a number of ways, such as sauna exposure and hot water immersion. Passive HA can induce physiological adaptation and may improve exercise performance (14;15), but direct comparisons between active and passive hyperthermia are lacking. Taylor (2) suggested that active HA may be superior to passive because a greater thermal strain could be experienced (exercise plus warm/hot ambient conditions rather than warm/hot ambient conditions alone). Undertaking passive HA (40 min per day of warm (40°C) water immersion for six days) immediately following exercise in cool conditions (18°C) can induce beneficial physiological and perceptual adaptations to the heat and improve running performance (16), and so "train cool, bathe hot" appears to be a practical HA option.

6.2.4.5 Can you acclimate to the heat by wearing more layers?

One area that is beginning to receive some attention is the idea that overdressing (i.e. wearing additional clothing while exercise) could mimic hot ambient conditions and provide a practical heat stress option (17–19). When looking at the acute effect of overdressing, it has been shown that 80 min of moderate cycling in temperate conditions (~17°C and ~82% relative humidity) with additional clothing (full-length spandex pants and a "winter" cycling jacket and gloves) elevates physiological (mean core body temperature and heart rate) and perceptual strain (thermal sensation and thermal comfort) compared to wearing just spandex shorts and a short sleeve top (19). In a similar study, runners asked to run submaximally for 60 min wearing a lot of additional clothing (two mid-weight wicking long-sleeved t-shirts, a long-sleeved shirt, a coat with heat-retaining lining, a waterproof rain jacket, a fleece hat, mittens, fitted short running tights, long mid-weight running tights, long loose-fit track pants, waterproof rain pants, and socks) had greater rates of rise in core body temperature, higher sweat rates, and greater extracellular heat-shock protein expression than when they undertook the same exercise wearing a sleeveless running singlet and lightweight running shorts (18). Unlike in the study conducted by Stevens et al. (19), heart rate was not different between the trials in men (somewhat surprising considering the greater thermal strain) but it was elevated by the overclothing in the female participants. In the only HA study to investigate overdressing, seven days of interval treadmill running in hot, humid conditions while wearing normal athletic gear (shorts, socks, and shoes) was compared against doing the same exercise in cool conditions while dressed in shorts, socks and t-shirt, polyester cotton tracksuit, cotton lined 100% nylon spray-proof pants and jacket, and an acrylic cloth bobble hat (17). The mean skin temperature was similar during the training sessions for both groups (~35°C), suggesting that the overdressing created a similar thermal stress to the warm conditions, and both groups acclimated to the heat (lower core body temperature, skin temperature, and heart rate following the intervention).

These data suggest that overdressing while exercising in cool conditions may be an effective and practical alternative to HA protocols; however, overdressing may not be as thermally demanding as more traditional approaches and so other ways of increasing the physiological strain (e.g. exercising at a higher intensity, wearing even more clothes, and/or exercising with more clothes in warmer conditions) should be considered. Consideration should also be made for the potential hobbling effect of exercising in extra clothing (e.g. limb movement could be impaired if lots of layers were worn during running).

6.3 The effect of HA on exercise performance

A recent meta-analysis reviewed 96 research articles and concluded that HA has a moderately beneficial effect on subsequent exercise capacity and performance in the heat irrespective of regimen (4). The mean improvement is +15% but there is a large range (standard deviation ± 22%) and so the median may be the more appropriate average – the median benefit on exercise performance is +6% with a range from no improvement (0%) to a very large improvement (+92%). Exercise capacity tests are open-ended (i.e., they have no predetermined end point and athletes are asked to exercise to volitional exhaustion) and as a result are more variable than performance tests that have a fixed finish point. Therefore, unsurprisingly, due to the open-ended nature of the test, capacity tests have greater improvements (mean: +23 ± 29%; median: +8 (0–92) %) than performance tests (mean: +7 ± 7%; median: +4 (0–33) %) following HA.

The benefit to exercise performance and capacity is related to the frequency, duration, and heat stress intensity of the HA protocol used; thus, when it comes to HA as a way of improving exercise performance in the heat, it is a case of the more the exposure, the better. Although protocols with 15+ HA sessions (LTHA) tend to have the greatest HA duration, some STHA protocols have a greater total heat exposure duration than some of the LTHA alternatives despite only involving a maximum of seven heat exposures. The exercise performance and capacity benefit observed following HA are similar between LTHA (mean: +22 ± 29%; median: +10 (4–65) %) and

MTHA (mean: +21 ± 28%; median: +9 (1–92) %) with both approaches being more effective than STHA (mean: +7 ± 8%; median: +4 (0–33) %) regimens. Performance data are seldom recorded part-way during a HA intervention, and so it is difficult to establish the time course of adaptation, but one paper that did report such data (20) reported that cycling performance was improved following six days of HA (STHA), and further improved after 14 days (MTHA). These data support the suggesting that where possible HA regimens should be as long as possible.

The isothermic HA approach is often purported to be the optimal one because it can continue to provide a thermal impulse to facilitate adaptation but there appears to be very little difference between the constant work (Hedges' g = 0.63 (0.46–0.79)) and isothermic approaches (Hedges' g = 0.63 (0.20–1.07)) with both approaches having a moderately beneficial effect on subsequent exercise performance or capacity. Interestingly, based upon the reviewed literature, both approaches are less effective than the self-regulated work approach (Hedges' g = 1.12 (0.78–1.45)) despite the potential for a suboptimal intensity to be self-selected. This potential issue seems to be overcome by the recruitment of well-motivated athletes who appear to self-select a sufficiently high enough intensity (20;21). Performance data are lacking for passive isothermal investigations but fixed-duration passive HA may be beneficial (16). Zurawlew et al. (16) reported that 5 km time-trial performance in hot ambient conditions (33°C) was improved by ~5% (Hedges' g = 0.40 (−0.49–1.28)) by bathing in warm water (40°C) for 40 min on six consecutive days immediately after 40 min of exercise in temperate conditions (18°C). This approach offers a potentially practical HA option for athletes with limited resources.

6.4 The physiological and perceptual responses to heat adaptation

Sawka et al. (22) stated that there were four "classic markers of heat adaptation":

1. A lower heart rate
2. A lower core body temperature
3. A higher sweat rate
4. An improved exercise performance in hot conditions

While these are all key indicators of heat adaptation, complete adaptation is wider-ranging. In addition to these four physiological variables, complete adaptation to heat also requires positive changes in other variables such as stroke volume, sodium loss, urine loss, water loss, skin blood flow, mean arterial pressure, central venous pressure, blood volume, and plasma osmolality (2) (Figure 6.2). Figure 6.3 highlights the effect that HA regimens of various frequencies can have on some of the key markers of adaptation.

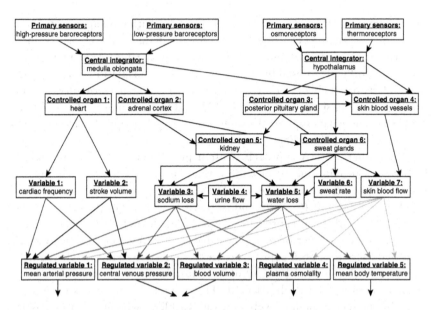

FIGURE 6.2 An integrated overview of heat adaptation. Reproduced from Taylor (2) with permission from John Wiley and Sons. Copyright 2014 American Physiological Society.

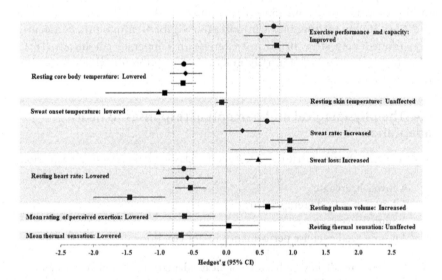

FIGURE 6.3 Forest plot summarising the effect [± 95% confidence intervals] of heat adaptation on exercise performance and capacity, and on key physiological and perceptual responses. Circle marker = effect size from all HA studies; diamond marker = effect size from STHA studies; square marker = effect size from MTHA studies; and triangle marker = effect size from LTHA studies. Solid line (Hedges' g = 0.0) = no effect. Modified from Tyler et al. (4).

6.4.1 Effect of HA on core body and skin temperature

HA reduces resting, mean, and comparable time-point core body temperature (4). The majority of core body temperature adaptations occur within the first seven days of HA with minimal difference between the adaptations observed following STHA and MTHA (~0.17°C reduction) (4). Further adaptations can be achieved if the thermal impulse is maintained as demonstrated by Patterson et al. (23) who maintained the thermal impulse by using an isothermal model and reported that core body temperature was 0.20°C lower after eight days of HA but 0.32°C lower after 22 days.

HA does not lower resting skin temperature but it can lower the mean skin temperature during exercise (4). The lower skin temperature may be due to an earlier skin blood flow response following HA because although the data are limited, it seems that HA causes the increase in skin blood flow to occur earlier (4). This earlier movement of blood to the periphery would facilitate the earlier transfer of heat from the core and increase evaporative heat loss (24) by increasing the cutaneous water vapour pressure at the skin.

6.4.2 Effect of HA on cardiovascular stability

The increase in peripheral blood flow during heat exposure helps to attenuate the thermoregulatory strain experienced by facilitating heat loss; however, it also places the body under greater cardiovascular strain (25). Fortunately, HA lowers resting and mean heart rate (4) and the heart rate adaptations to heat are some of the first to be observed following HA. As with core body temperature changes, the effects of STHA and MTHA on lowering resting heart rate are similar (4) which suggests that most of the heart rate adaptations occur within the first week of HA. Heart rate adaptations can continue past seven days if the thermal impulse is maintained; for example, Patterson et al. (23) reported that resting heart rate was reduced by 5 b·min^{-1} after eight days of isothermic HA and by an additional 5 b·min^{-1} after 22 days of isothermic HA.

Blood pressure, stroke volume, and cardiac output are also modulated by HA with reductions or maintenance in systolic (26–29), diastolic (26–29), and mean (27;30;31) arterial pressures, lower cardiac output (32), and increased stroke volume (32–35) reported; however, fewer studies have reported such data. The heat-induced changes in cardiac variables occur largely due to increases in plasma volume (hypervolemia) which are observed following HA regardless of regimen. The mean (+4.3 ± 4.7%) and median (+3%) increases following HA are similar; however, a wide range of PV changes have been reported (−1.9 to +16%) (4). Different HA approaches appear to explain much of this variation with constant work protocols seeing a short-lived improvement (35) and isothermic protocols reporting sustained plasma volume expansion (36).

6.4.3 Effect of HA on sweat responses

HA can markedly reduce the sudomotor threshold (i.e. the onset temperature at which sweating commences) and can elevate sweat sensitivity, sweat rate, and total sweat loss. LTHA has the greatest effect on increasing total sweat loss and although STHA approaches can elevate sweat rate, large increases are only observed following MTHA and LTHA (4). Sweat response adaptations may take up to one month to be complete (37) and there is a strong, positive relationship between the effect size reported for sweat rate and the duration of the HA regimen, which suggests that more is more! The sweat response appears to be driven, at least in part (38), by the magnitude of change in core body temperature because the magnitudes of reduction observed in resting core and sweat onset temperatures (sudomotor threshold) are very similar ($-0.24°C$ versus $-0.26°C$) (24;39–41). An aligned reduction would be beneficial because it would allow evaporative heat loss to start at a lower core body temperature and may reduce the magnitude of thermal strain experienced. Increases in sweat loss (i.e. sudomotor capacity) only benefit the athlete if heat can be lost. As mentioned in Chapter 2, the evaporation of sweat is the primary heat loss pathway during exercise in the heat and so to be beneficial, an increase in sweat loss needs to be matched with an increase in evaporative heat loss. HA increases an athlete's evaporative capacity by ~11% (24;42), but this increase is only a third of the increase in HA-induced sweat production (~30%) and so there is a ~200% increase in the amount of unevaporated sweat (42). This may offer a benefit to humid-heat adaptation (43), but due to the disparity in adaptations, they are unlikely to augment the magnitude of thermal strain experienced and perceived in the heat in hot, dry conditions.

As well as altering the sweat response, HA can alter the sweat concentration. If you exercise in the heat and start sweating, you might start to taste salt – this is because sweat naturally contains electrolytes such as sodium and chloride (these make up table salt and so it is unsurprising that sweat tastes salty). HA enhances the reabsorption of these electrolytes resulting in lower sweat concentrations of sodium and chloride and more dilute sweat – so in theory, if you exercise regularly in the heat, your sweat should taste less and less salty as you adapt to the stress. A more dilute sweat is advantageous because due to the lower cutaneous water vapour pressure it can be more readily evaporated (2).

6.4.4 Effect of HA on markers of fluid balance

Limited data exist but what does exist suggest that HA may decrease the sensation of thirst (44–46) and volitional fluid consumption (20; 44–47); however, both increases (20;47) and decreases (44–46) in volitional fluid consumption have been observed. If thirst is a key driver of fluid consumption (see Chapter 8 for more detail on thirst), a decrease in thirst sensation should decrease volitional fluid consumption. This may lead to a state of hypohydration and so prescribed fluid regimens may be needed (see Chapter 8 for more information on the effect of hypohydration on the body, exercise, and cognitive performance).

6.4.5 Effect of HA on ratings of perceived exertion and thermal sensation

A reduction in the perceived exertion and improved thermal sensations and comfort (see Chapter 3 for more detail on these topics) would likely be beneficial to an athlete because reductions in perceived exertion should enable individuals to self-select a higher intensity during performance (closed-loop) events and exercise for longer in capacity (open-loop) tests, because thermal sensation and thermal comfort are key drivers of volitional behaviour. Data are only available from a very small number of studies, and so should be interpreted with caution, but the available data suggest that HA can reduce the mean ratings of perceived exertion (26;48;49) and thermal sensation (49–51) reported during exercise. Thermal comfort seems to track seasonal variations in air temperature (i.e. hot temperatures are better tolerated in the summer months) (52), which suggests that some natural heat acclimatisation can occur without any specific intention to make it happen.

6.4.6 Molecular basis to HA

When an organism is exposed to repeated bout of heat exposure, a heat-shock response is triggered and these responses are often classified by the expression site and molecular mass of the proteins expressed – the most commonly reported proteins in the heat adaptation literature are heat-shock proteins 72 and 90 (the number denotes the molecular mass). Heat-shock proteins within the cell (intracellular heat-shock proteins) regulate protein structure while those outside of the cell (extracellular heat-shock proteins) appear to have an anti-inflammatory function (53). Essentially, intra- and extra-cellular heat-shock proteins serve to improve the stability of the cell when subjected to future heat strain and this is often referred to as increased/improved thermotolerance. The extent of the heat-shock protein expression is dependent upon the magnitude of heat strain (54) and so greater disturbances to thermal homeostasis result in greater expression. Extracellular concentrations of heat-shock proteins are largely unaffected by HA (4) but, in contrast, concentrations of intracellular heat-shock protein 72 appear to be markedly increased by HA with increases of up to 320% reported (54). The molecular response to HA is a relatively new area of research and so there are limited data. More research is required to elucidate the effects of HA on the human heat-shock response and establish the practical meaning of any such response, so if your department has the facilities, there are many potential research questions you could pick from.

6.5 Cross-adaptation: HA for performance in other conditions

It has been proposed that acclimation to one environmental stressor may result in adaptations beneficial in another (e.g. adaptations made in response to a HA regimen may be beneficial in hypoxic – this has been called "cross adaptation" or "cross-tolerance").

Quick question: In order for adaptations to one environmental stressor (e.g. heat) to be beneficial in another (e.g. cooler conditions or those with low oxygen availability), the adaptations must be mutually beneficial. From what you now know about the physiological adaptations to heat acclimation, which do you think may benefit (or hinder) performance in cooler conditions or conditions with low oxygen concentrations?

6.5.1 Temperate and cooler conditions

There is debate whether there is a benefit of HA on exercise performance in cooler conditions but as discussed in Chapter 4, core body temperature can increase during exercise in cooler conditions and this can place a sufficient thermal strain to limit performance. Galloway and Maughan (55) reported that exercise capacity is impaired in conditions above 11°C – a relatively cool temperature – and so adaptations may be beneficial when exercising in conditions warmer than this. It seems likely that the greatest benefit would be observed in conditions that result in the greatest thermal strain and so any benefit is likely to reduce as the thermal stress decreases.

Improved exercise performance in cooler conditions after a period of HA has been reported (32; 53; 56; 57). HA has been reported to improve mean peak power output in an incremental cycling exercise test by ~4% (28) and Yo-Yo shuttle test distance by 7–44% (56;57;51) in cooler conditions (21–23°C); however, the lack of appropriate control groups in most studies means that the data are somewhat equivocal. Some investigations reported a benefit 30 days after HA (having not observed one ten days after) which is interesting because this time frame does not match the typical time course for HA decay and suggests that the ergogenic effect may be due to other, unreported, factors. Lorenzo et al. (32) conducted a study (with a control group which undertook the same exercise in cooler conditions) and reported that not only did HA induce beneficial physiological adaptations and improve exercise performance under the hot conditions, but also increased the amount of work completed in a 60 min cycling test by ~ 6% under cool (13°C) conditions. The data from Lorenzo et al. (32) and others suggest that there might be a benefit of HA to exercise performed in cooler condition but more research is required.

A number of physiological adaptations to HA could potentially offer a benefit to exercise performance in cooler conditions – these include lower core body and skin temperatures at a given intensity, lower heart rate, increased economy, increased maximal oxygen uptake, plasma volume expansion, and an increased lactate threshold (32;58). Plasma volume expansion caused by HA can increase cardiac output in cooler conditions (32) (possibly due to an increased stroke volume), and this increased cardiac output may lead to improved cardiac stability and lower heart rates, and may explain the increased maximal oxygen uptake observed in cool conditions following HA (32;58), although the effect of hypervolemia on maximal oxygen uptake in trained populations is a controversial topic at present. The effects of other HA-induced adaptation in cooler conditions are less clear. For example, HA modulates the sweat response, increasing the sweat rate and causing the sweat onset to occur earlier – if this occurred in conditions which were too cool, the athlete could potentially lose heat too early and begin to feel uncomfortably cold. The topic of cross-acclimation is a relatively new one and so an area for future research.

6.5.2 Hypoxia

While the transfer of HA adaptations to cooler conditions may seem logical due to temperature being a common feature, it has also been proposed that HA adaptations may be beneficial in high altitude/hypoxic environments. The main factor that limits exercise in hypoxic conditions is a reduced oxygen delivery and utilisation and although not a major limiting factor in the heat, both heat stress and hypoxia compromise oxygen delivery to the working muscle (albeit via different pathways).

Although data are limited, it appears that HA adaptations can improve exercise performance in hypoxic conditions by ~ 2–5% (50;59). In one study, participants completed a self-paced 16.1 km time trial in hypoxic conditions 2 min (4.8%) quicker following HA (50), whereas in the other hypoxic time trial, performance was improved by 28 s by ten days of HA (1,745 s versus 1,722 s) – a 1.6% improvement (59).

The adaptations that may explain this enhanced performance in other environmental extremes are likely to be multifactorial and occurring at the whole-body and cellular levels. HA can reduce the physiological strain observed during hypoxic exposure – namely by reducing heart rate (50;60), increasing oxygen saturation (50;60), and even reducing skin and core body temperatures (50). Despite the lower thermal strain (50), the improved performance is most likely to be explained by the cardiovascular, rather than thermoregulatory, adaptations (unless the hypoxic stress is present alongside a thermal one (e.g. if insulative clothing is worn at altitude during periods of intense exercise or work)). The key cardiovascular adaptation to HA which may have a benefit in hypoxic conditions is one of the adaptations discussed in the section regarding cross-adaptation for cooler conditions – hypervolemia. A HA-induced plasma volume expansion may be beneficial at altitude as it is able to help maintain cardiac output and oxygen delivery. The increased oxygen delivery may be further aided by cellular adaptations – namely the expression of hypoxia-inducible factor 1-alpha (HIF-1 α) during the course of HA. HIF-1 α is involved in processes such as angiogenesis (the growth of blood vessels from the existing vasculature) and erythropoiesis (the production of new red blood cells), both of which can improve the oxygen delivery to potentially hypoxic tissues (61). Although HIF-1 α is more commonly discussed when talking about adaptations to hypoxic conditions, it is expressed as a result of both hypoxic and thermal strain and interestingly its stability is improved by the expression of heat-shock proteins. There appears to be an overlap of physiological and cellular responses to heat and hypoxic stress and so it seems prudent to suggest that there may be a beneficial molecular crossover between the environmental stressors. As with the cross-adaptation for cooler conditions, the topic of whether HA can offer a benefit to hypoxic conditions is a new and developing one. HA is often easier to undertake than hypoxic acclimation and so cross-acclimation would be useful to athletes about to compete in conditions of low oxygen; however, more data are required before recommendations to athletes can be made.

6.6 HA decay

Despite there being many research articles focusing on HA, there are far fewer looking at HA decay (sometimes called heat deacclimation). It stands to reason that if the heat adaptation trigger (i.e. a thermal impulse that exceeds the adaptation threshold (2)) is removed, athletes are no longer exposed to regular heat exposure that the adaptations to the hot conditions will be lost as the athletes begin to adapt to the new, cooler temperatures faced.

The magnitude of decay can be calculated in absolute (e.g. °C increase) or relative terms – relative terms have recently been proposed as the preferable approach (62). Relative HA decay can be expressed as a percentage and calculated as follows:

- % HA decay = 100 × (acclimated value – value after decay)/(acclimated value – unacclimated value)

For example, if resting heart rate is 64 b·min^{-1} before HA, 58 b·min^{-1} after ten days of HA, and then 62 b·min^{-1} seven days after HA, the relative decay can be calculated as follows:

%HA decay = $100 \times (58 - 62)/(58 - 64)$

%HA decay = $100 \times -4/-6$

%HA decay = 100×0.667

%HA decay = 66.7%

(*i.e.* second / third of heat adaptation has been lost at a rate of 9.5% per day)

6.6.1 Decay in heart rate adaptations

The fictional rate of decay above (~9.5% per day) is ~4 × greater than the real rate with Daanen et al. (62) estimating that although decay in heart rate adaptation does not always occur, heart rate adaptations to heat are lost at an average rate of ~2.3% per day. It appears that the decay is progressive over time but it is not clear how soon it can be observed. Poirier et al. (24) reported a relative heart rate HA decay of ~40% (5.7% per day) and ~53% (3.8% per day) one week and two weeks after HA, respectively, whereas neither Ashley et al. (63) nor Garrett et al. (64) reported any decay within the first week following HA. Garrett et al. (64)

reported that there was an average decay of 31% after two weeks (2.2% per day) and 54% after three weeks (2.6% per day) whereas Ashley et al. (63) reported that all adaptations were lost after three weeks. Daanen et al. (62) reported that the decay in heart rate can be predicted using the following equation:

Heart rate decay$(\%) = 3.6 + 2.3 \times$ number of decay days

6.6.2 Decay in core body temperature adaptations

Due to relatively small changes observed during the preceding HA regimens reviewed, Daanen et al. (62) reported a very large range in the decay in core body temperature adaptations with very large losses (−246% (65)) and gains (+180% (64)) observed. The largest decay was observed because large reductions in core body temperature (−0.3°C) occurred after, not during, the HA protocol (65). Relative decay in core body temperature adaptations is similarly variable. Garrett et al. (64) and Pandolf et al. (7) reported HA decay in core body temperature of 1.1% per day, whereas Poirier et al. (24) and Pichan et al. (66) saw a relative decay of 3.1% per day and 2.0% per day two and three weeks after HA, respectively. As with the decay of heart rate adaptations, the decay appears progressive. Stephens and Hoag (67) reported that the mean decay in core body temperature adaptations was 40%, 44%, and 60%, 5, 17, and 33 days after HA meaning that the adaptations were lost at a slow rate − 8.0%, 2.6%, and 1.8% per day.

The decay in core body temperature adaptations can be predicted using the following regression equation produced by Daanen et al. (62) which involves three items − the number of days without HA (decay days), the duration of the daily heat exposure, and the heat stress of the session expressed at wet-bulb globe temperature:

Decay in core body temperature adaptations to heat$(\%) = -126 + 2.6$
$\times$ number of decay days $- 1.2 \times$ HA duration $+ 6.8 \times$ HA temperature

This regression equation indicates that the loss of core body temperature adaptations is slow (~2.6% per day) and that longer, less stressful reacclimation sessions can slow the rate of decay.

6.6.3 Decay in sweat response adaptations

The mean reduction in sweat rate adaptations is approximately 21% although there is also a large range in decay for this variable (62). Most studies report a fairly rapid decay in sweat rate adaptation with 26–175% lost within the first week following HA and 63–175% lost two or more weeks after (65;66;68;69). Daanen et al. (62) reported that sweat response adaptation decay could be estimated using the following equation but they advised caution because only seven studies were used to produce the equation:

Decay in sweat rate adaptations to heat $(\%) = 964 - 27.7 \times$ number of HA days $- 18.2 \times$ HA temperature

Highly thermally stressful conditions during HA appear to sow the rate of decay in sweat response adaptations, and so if sweat adaptations are particularly important, this should be considered when designing the HA protocol.

6.6.4 Decay in performance improvements

HA performance benefits may last 1–2 weeks post HA but the data are very limited. Ashley et al. (63) reported that exercise capacity was similar immediately (115 min) and three weeks (116 min) post HA although in this study only a few participants failed to complete the entire 120 min bout and so the differences were only minor. Similarly consistent data were observed by Daanen et al. who reported that exercise capacity following nine days of HA (capacity time = 46.5 min) was almost identical seven days later following HA (46.4 min) suggesting that performance benefits can last at least one week (65). In contrast, Garrett et al. (64) reported that HA successfully improved exercise performance when comparing pre- and post-performance data (12.4 versus 14.2 min), but that the benefit began to decline one week after HA (13.7 min) and that the decline was greater still two weeks after (12.7 min).

6.7 Heat reacclimation

Although heat adaptations decay, it has been shown that the rate of adaptation is faster when reacclimating to heat which could be very useful to a time-short athlete. A number of reacclimation approaches have been investigated with many using only 2–3 days of heat reacclimation (HR) (63;66–68;70–72). Heart rate reductions are one of the earliest observed adaptations to heat but HR appears to be even more efficient at lowering heart rate (63;66–68;70;72). A faster rate of adaptation may occur because some of the initial adaptations are retained; however, HR may also actually induce greater adaptations than HA. Saat et al. (68) reported that heart rate was lower after 14 days of HA but it was even lower at the end of 10 days of HR, and Lind and Bass (71) also reported that heart rate and core body temperature reductions after five days of HR were greater than after HA. HR appears to be about eight times stronger than HA decay for inducing heart rate adaptations, which means that a month of HA decay might be compensated by only about four days of HR (67).

Core body temperature adaptations can also occur following a period of HR and these adaptations might be even quicker than the cardiovascular ones. Weller et al. (72) reported that two days of HR can compensate for 26 days of HA decay for heart rate adaptations but that only one day of HR was required to return core body temperature to HA levels after 26 days of HA decay. With this in mind, whereas HR is about eight times stronger than HA decay for reversing heart rate changes, HR is about 12 times stronger than HA decay for reversing loses in core body temperature adaptations.

Overall, it appears that two weeks of HA decay will reduce heart rate, core body temperature, and sweat rate adaptations by approximately 35, 6, and 30%, respectively, if full adaptation occurs (62) but all of the decay can be reversed if HR is undertaken for 4–5 days (62).

Problem 6.1 revisited: Heat acclimation on a budget

You are a volunteer coach for a local Scottish football team that has been invited to take part in a summer tournament in Barcelona. The temperature is forecast to be 30–35°C and you would like to prepare the team for the heat prior to flying out because your first match is scheduled to take place 24 h after you land in Barcelona. You and the team fly out in 14 days so you have time to prepare but unfortunately you do not have access to an environmental chamber and the local temperatures are not expected to exceed 20°C. What can you do to prepare your athletes for the heat that is inexpensive and does not require any specialist equipment?

You have three main things to consider before putting together a plan:

1. Can you acclimatise?
2. What resources do you have?
3. How long do you have?

Unfortunately, acclimatising is not an option for two reasons – the local temperatures are not going to exceed 20°C, and you are only arriving in Barcelona 24 h before the first match. You can ensure that your players experience the environmental conditions in Barcelona in the time between landing and playing but your players are not going to make any meaningful physiological adaptations in a single day.

You do not have access to an environmental chamber but there are other ways that you can create a thermally stressful environment. What are they? You could either use regular heaters to heat a room or you could ask the athletes to wear more clothes than normal when exercising. Heating the room would simulate the high temperatures nicely and although it is more difficult to create a humid environment it is possible. A number of years ago, I was a participant for a research project investigating the sweat responses to cycling in the heat; the room was a normal room heated with regular portable heaters, and humidity was created by boiling water on a travel stove and in a number of kettles spaced around the room! If heating a room is not possible (e.g. you want to undertake your usual football-based training and require a football pitch), as discussed earlier, overdressing is a practical alternative to provide a heat stress. The stress provided might not match that faced in Barcelona (17–19), but some HA is better than none, and with two weeks' worth of heat stress, adaptations would be expected. The other option available to you is to instruct your players to have a hot bath after training in normal conditions. Body temperature will be elevated by the exercise and a daily 40-min warm (40°C) bath immediately after exercise (even in cool conditions (18°C)) can induce beneficial physiological and perceptual adaptations to the heat and improve running performance (16).

Problem 6.2 revisited: Optimising heat acclimation for the elite athlete

You are the head physiologist for the National Athletic Association and planning for an upcoming competition in a foreign country where the temperatures are expected to exceed 30°C. You have been instructed to develop a four-week plan to help the marathon runners deal with the conditions. Your athletes will arrive at the competition one week before it is due to start but fortunately your domestic training facility has an environmental chamber on site. What will you do?

In this example, if we ask ourselves the same three questions as before, the answers will be very different.

1. Can you acclimatise?

    Yes, you can. Your athletes are flying out seven days in advance of the competition and so will be able to acclimatise to the exact conditions (unless the weather suddenly changes!)
2. What resources do you have?

    In addition to being able to acclimatise, you have access to an environmental chamber which allows you to have a tight control over the conditions you ask your athletes to train and acclimate in.
3. How long do you have?

    You have been asked to devise a four-week plan, and so have three weeks before you fly out to acclimate your athletes and one week to acclimatise your athletes in the country where the competition will take place.

There are a number of factors that will need to be considered when designing the preparation plan (e.g. training schedules and media commitments) but you have been asked to focus on designing a four-week plan to help the athletes cope with the forecasted hot conditions so we will focus on this aspect. As discussed in Chapter 4, longer duration events are more impacted on by the heat than shorter, more explosive activities and so it is great that you have a whole month to prepare as most of the desired adaptations will occur in this time frame with an effective HA regimen.

Consecutive days or not? By having so long, you are able to design a LTHA protocol involving more than 15 exposures. Four weeks gives you 28 days and so you could have 28 consecutive days of heat exposure; however, this might be impractical (or even unadvisable due to the risk of overtraining) and so it is important to remember that heat adaptation still occurs if HA sessions take place every 2–3 days (5). If consecutive days were used, you may wish to combine active and passive HA because passive HA can also induce beneficial physiological adaptations to high temperatures and may improve exercise performance (14;15). If a break from the HA is required, all is not lost because any heat adaptation decay can be reversed with 4–5 days of HR (62).

How long should each session last? There is little consensus on the optimal duration of each HA session but current recommendations suggest at least 60 min a day (6) and due to the requirements of the marathon training durations exceeding this are likely to be common anyway.

How thermally stressful should the environment be? Physiological adaptations and improved exercise performance are moderately linked to the temperature used which suggests that more adaptations occur at hotter temperatures. You need to ensure that your athletes adapt to the temperatures expected (>30°C) but have the time to do that gradually. In order to strike a balance between being able to maintain training and adapting to the heat, I suggest a progressive increase in the thermal stress over the course of the three weeks in the environmental chamber so that the athletes are well prepared for their week acclimatising at the venue. If for some reason the environmental chamber cannot be used, remember that stress can be caused by wearing additional clothing during exercise (17–19).

How intense should the sessions be? Most often prolonged, sub-maximal exercise is used. Data which directly compare HA of different intensities are scarce and although higher intensity HA is receiving some attention, it is largely for time-short situations. You have four weeks, so normal training intensities are most likely to be fine and should minimise the risk of overtraining (12).

What type of HA protocol should you use? The constant work method is frequently used because it is logistically easier to acclimate a number of athletes simultaneously; however, it is difficult to ensure that the thermal impulse is sufficient for adaptation using this approach. The isothermic/controlled hyperthermia acclimation approach overcomes this shortcoming but requires close monitoring of physiological strain to ensure that a constant overload is applied. Typically, this involves the measurement of core body temperature but because this may be logistically challenging, heart rate monitoring has been recommended. Monitoring your athletes is a very good idea to assess whether adaptation is occurring but if it is not possible then the isothermic HA approach is impossible. Fortunately, well-motivated athletes appear to self-select an intensity sufficient to result in adaptations (4), and so the athletes should be okay self-regulating their intensity. As they begin to get used to the heat, the intensity should naturally increase maintaining the thermal impulse.

6.8 Summary

HA and acclimatisation can be highly effective at reducing physiological and perceptual strain in hot environmental conditions and may improve exercise performance as a result. Successful HA can cause many beneficial physiological and perceptual adaptations to high ambient temperatures, but the time course of adaptation is variable-specific. The majority of core body temperature and heart rate adaptations occur within the first seven days of HA (4), although further adaptations can be achieved if the thermal impulse is maintained (23). Sweat responses generally take longer to be observed with LTHA having the greatest effect on increasing total sweat loss (4), and sweat response adaptations may take up to one month to be complete (37). A number of adaptations to heat could potentially benefit exercise performed in other environmental extremes and limited data suggest that HA may indeed improve exercise performance in cooler (32; 51;56;57) and hypoxic (50;59) conditions but more research is required.

While the *average* HA protocol involves nine consecutive HA sessions each lasting 105 min of exercise in hot conditions (40°C, 40% relative humidity) (4), the actual protocols used vary considerably, and there is little consensus on what makes for an optimal programme. STHA (<7 exposures), MTHA (8–14 exposures), and LTHA (> 15 exposures) approaches have been used. The optimal HA duration, heat stress intensity, and exercise intensity are likely to be sport and situational specific with athletes advised to acclimate to the specific environmental conditions likely to be faced using sport-specific intensities and activity patterns. When selecting the HA approach, one of three HA types can be used – self-regulated/self-paced work HA; constant work HA; or isothermic/controlled hyperthermia HA. The self-regulated work and constant work models may provide an insufficient thermal impulse to cause adaptations due to the non-specific approach; however, this may not be a problem for well-motivated participants who may self-select an intensity sufficient to cause adaptation (4). In order to have greater control over the thermal impulse provided (and to ensure that the strain is progressively greater), the isothermic HA model has been increasingly used. This approach can be active or passive and aims to elevate core body temperature to a target core body temperature (often 38.5°C).

The rate of HA decay is variable between studies and between variables, but heart rate and core body temperature adaptations to heat appear to be lost at an average rate of approximately 2–3% per day (62). HA performance benefits may last 1–2 weeks post HA but the data are very limited. Interestingly, following a period of HA decay, the rate of HR is quicker than if no previous HA had been completed, and all of the decay can be reversed if HR is undertaken for only 4–5 days (62).

If heat adaptation is desired, athletes should:

1. Spend as much time as possible exposed to high ambient temperatures.
2. Ideally, start exercising in hot conditions at least 14 days prior to the event – this could either take the form of HA, heat acclimatisation, or a combination of both.
3. Undertake active, rather than passive, HA.
4. Expose themselves to ambient conditions that mimic the expected conditions.
5. Undertake consecutive days of HA if possible; however, heat exposure every other, or every third, day can still induce beneficial adaptations.

In order to facilitate effective and safe heat adaptation, coaches should:

1. Monitor and progressively increase exercise intensity to ensure that over-loading and adaptation continue to occur.
2. Monitor the athletes closely. While core body temperature is preferable, HR may be a practical way to ensure an appropriate magnitude of physiological strain during HA when the measurement of core body temperature is impractical. Heat adaptation would be expected to lower HR at any given intensity.
3. Be aware that due to reductions in work capacity in the heat, the heat stress needs to be progressively increased – this could be by exercising in progressively hotter conditions (e.g. different times of the day) and/or progressively increasing the intensity of exercise bouts

6.9 Self-check quiz

At the beginning of this chapter you were told that by this point you should know the following:

- What is the difference between heat acclimation and heat acclimatisation? Do the different approaches have different effects on exercise performance and the physiological responses to exercise in the heat?
- The different heat adaptation protocols used and what their strengths and weaknesses are
- Differences between active and passive heat acclimation
- Physiological, perceptual, and molecular responses to heat acclimation
- Whether heat adaptation can offer a benefit in other environmental extremes
- The rate and extent of heat acclimation decay
- Heat reacclimation and decay considerations

The quick self-check quiz below will help you determine whether you have learnt the relevant material. You may need to revisit the chapter in order to help you – this is fine and encouraged!

6.9.1 Self-check quiz questions

1. What is the difference between heat acclimation and heat adaptation when defining the heat adaptation approach used?
2. In order to adapt to hot environmental conditions, what does the thermal impulse(s) need to exceed?
3. Medium-term heat acclimation comprises of how many heat exposures?
4. In what four main ways can a heat adaptation regimen differ from another?
5. What are the three most commonly used heat acclimation regimen types?
6. What are the four classic markers of heat adaptation as identified by Sawka (22)?
7. It has been proposed that heat adaptation may be beneficial in other environments (e.g. cold and hypoxia) – what is this phenomenon referred to as?
8. How can you calculate the percentage of heat acclimation decay?
9. How long lasting are the benefits of heat acclimation on exercise performance?
10. How much more efficient is heat reacclimation than heat acclimation decay?

6.9.2 Self-check quiz answers

1. Heat acclimation describes artificially induced heat adaptation (e.g. using a laboratory-based environmental chamber), whereas heat acclimatisation describes adaptations induced by natural exposure (e.g. warm-weather training camps or domestic exposure to elevated ambient temperatures).
2. An adaptation threshold.

3. 8–14.
4. The frequency of exposures, the duration of exposure, the intensity of the heat stress and strain, and the heat acclimation type used.
5. Self-regulated/self-paced work; constant work; isothermic/controlled hyperthermia.
6. Lower heart rate, lower core body temperature, higher sweat rate, and improved exercise performance in hot conditions.
7. Cross adaptation or cross tolerance.
8. % heat acclimation decay = 100 × (acclimated value − value after decay)/ (acclimated value − unacclimated value).
9. 1–2 weeks (although the data are limited).
10. Approximately eight times faster i.e. a month of heat acclimation decay might be compensated by only about four days of heat reacclimation.

6.10 Practical toolkit

TABLE 6.1 Different ways to acclimate/acclimatise

	Description	Pros	Cons
Self-regulated work	Individuals self-select the exercise intensity based upon their own perceived levels of discomfort caused by the heat exposure or other available cues	• Easy to deliver • No physiological monitoring is required • Effective for well-motivated participants who self-select an exercise intensity sufficient to result in adaptations	• The self-selected intensity may be insufficient to induce adaptation • It is difficult (sometimes impossible) to quantify the thermal strain experienced • Difficult to ensure that the progressive overload required for adaptation occurs
Constant work	Individuals work at a set intensity throughout the HA programme	• Easy and efficient to simultaneously acclimate multiple individuals to heat	• Unable to ensure that every athlete gets a sufficient thermal impulse for adaptation to occur
Controlled hyperthermia	Exercise and heat stress are manipulated to achieve a target core body temperature (often 38.5°C)	• Ensures a progressive thermal impulse is provided to facilitate adaptation • Can be active or passive	• Requires accurate core body temperature measurement • Requires specialist equipment

References

1 Glossary of terms for thermal physiology. 2nd ed. Revised by The Commission for Thermal Physiology of the International Union of Physiological Sciences (IUPS Thermal Commission). *Pflugers Arch* 1987 Nov;410(4–5):567–87.

2 Taylor NA. Human heat adaptation. *Compr Physiol* 2014 Jan;4(1):325–65.

3 Periard JD, Racinais S, Timpka T, Dahlstrom O, Spreco A, Jacobsson J, et al. Strategies and factors associated with preparing for competing in the heat: a cohort study at the 2015 IAAF World Athletics Championships. *Br J Sports Med* 2017 Feb;51(4):264–70.

4 Tyler CJ, Reeve T, Hodges GJ, Cheung SS. The effects of heat adaptation on physiology, perception and exercise performance in the heat: a meta-analysis. *Sports Med* 2016 Nov;46(11):1699–724.

5 Fein JT, Haymes EM, Buskirk ER. Effects of daily and intermittent exposures on heat acclimation of women. *Int J Biometeorol* 1975 Mar;19(1):41–52.

6 Racinais S, Alonso JM, Coutts AJ, Flouris AD, Girard O, Gonzalez-Alonso J, et al. Consensus recommendations on training and competing in the heat. *Sports Med* 2015 Jul;45(7):925–38.

7 Pandolf KB. Time course of heat acclimation and its decay. *Int J Sports Med* 1998 Jun;19 Suppl 2:S157–S160.

8 Houmard JA, Costill DL, Davis JA, Mitchell JB, Pascoe DD, Robergs RA. The influence of exercise intensity on heat acclimation in trained subjects. *Med Sci Sports Exerc* 1990 Oct;22(5):615–20.

9 Kelly M, Gastin PB, Dwyer DB, Sostaric S, Snow RJ. Short duration heat acclimation in Australian football players. *J Sports Sci Med* 2016 Mar;15(1):118–25.

10 Wingfield GL, Gale R, Minett GM, Marino FE, Skein M. The effect of high versus low intensity heat acclimation on performance and neuromuscular responses. *J Therm Biol* 2016 May;58:50–9.

11 Schmit C, Duffield R, Hausswirth C, Brisswalter J, Le MY. Optimizing heat acclimation for endurance athletes: high- vs low-intensity training. *Int J Sports Physiol Perform* 2017 Sep 5;1–24.

12 Kenefick RW, Maresh CM, Armstrong LE, Castellani JW, Whittlesey M, Hoffman JR, et al. Plasma testosterone and cortisol responses to training-intensity exercise in mild and hot environments. *Int J Sports Med* 1998 Apr;19(3):177–81.

13 Periard JD, Racinais S, Sawka MN. Adaptations and mechanisms of human heat acclimation: applications for competitive athletes and sports. *Scand J Med Sci Sports* 2015 Jun;25(Suppl. 1):20–38.

14 Pallubinsky H, Schellen L, Kingma BRM, Dautzenberg B, van Baak MA, van Marken Lichtenbelt WD. Thermophysiological adaptations to passive mild heat acclimation. *Temperature (Austin)* 2017;4(2):176–86.

15 Racinais S, Wilson MG, Periard JD. Passive heat acclimation improves skeletal muscle contractility in humans. *Am J Physiol Regul Integr Comp Physiol* 2017 Jan 1;312(1):R101–R107.

16 Zurawlew MJ, Walsh NP, Fortes MB, Potter C. Post-exercise hot water immersion induces heat acclimation and improves endurance exercise performance in the heat. *Scand J Med Sci Sports* 2016 Jul;26(7):745–54.

17 Dawson B, Pyke FS, Morton AR. Improvements in heat tolerance induced by interval running training in the heat and in sweat clothing in cool conditions. *J Sports Sci* 1989;7(3):189–203.

18 Ely BR, Blanchard LA, Steele JR, Francisco MA, Cheuvront SN, Minson CT. Physiological responses to overdressing and exercise-heat stress in trained runners. *Med Sci Sports Exerc* 2018 Jun;50(6):1285–96.

19 Stevens CJ, Plews DJ, Laursen PB, Kittel AB, Taylor L. Acute physiological and perceptual responses to wearing additional clothing while cycling outdoors in a temperate environment: a practical method to increase the heat load. *Temperature (Austin)* 2017;4(4):414–19.

20 Racinais S, Periard JD, Karlsen A, Nybo L. Effect of heat and heat acclimatization on cycling time trial performance and pacing. *Med Sci Sports Exerc* 2015 Mar;47(3):601–6.

21 Schmit C, Le MY, Duffield R, Robach P, Oussedik N, Coutts AJ, et al. Heat-acclimatization and pre-cooling: a further boost for endurance performance? *Scand J Med Sci Sports* 2017 Jan;27(1):55–65.

22 Sawka MN, Leon LR, Montain SJ, Sonna LA. Integrated physiological mechanisms of exercise performance, adaptation, and maladaptation to heat stress. *Compr Physiol* 2011 Oct;1(4):1883–928.

23 Patterson MJ, Stocks JM, Taylor NA. Humid heat acclimation does not elicit a preferential sweat redistribution toward the limbs. *Am J Physiol Regul Integr Comp Physiol* 2004 Mar;286(3):R512–R518.

24 Poirier MP, Gagnon D, Friesen BJ, Hardcastle SG, Kenny GP. Whole-body heat exchange during heat acclimation and its decay. *Med Sci Sports Exerc* 2015 Feb;47(2):390–400.

25 Gonzalez-Alonso J, Crandall CG, Johnson JM. The cardiovascular challenge of exercising in the heat. *J Physiol* 2008 Jan 1;586(1):45–53.

26 Armstrong LE, Maresh CM, Keith NR, Elliott TA, Vanheest JL, Scheett TP, et al. Heat acclimation and physical training adaptations of young women using different contraceptive hormones. *Am J Physiol Endocrinol Metab* 2005 May;288(5):E868–E875.

27 Maruyama M, Hara T, Hashimoto M, Koga M, Shido O. Alterations of calf venous and arterial compliance following acclimation to heat administered at a fixed daily time in humans. *Int J Biometeorol* 2006 May;50(5):269–74.

28 Poh PY, Armstrong LE, Casa DJ, Pescatello LS, McDermott BP, Emmanuel H, et al. Orthostatic hypotension after 10 days of exercise-heat acclimation and 28 hours of sleep loss. *Aviat Space Environ Med* 2012 Apr;83(4):403–11.

29 Shido O, Sakurada S, Sugimoto N, Hiratsuka Y, Takuwa Y. Ambient temperatures preferred by humans acclimated to heat given at a fixed daily time. *Physiol Behav* 2001 Feb;72(3):387–92.

30 Fujii N, Honda Y, Ogawa T, Tsuji B, Kondo N, Koga S, et al. Short-term exercise-heat acclimation enhances skin vasodilation but not hyperthermic hyperpnea in humans exercising in a hot environment. *Eur J Appl Physiol* 2012 Jan;112(1):295–307.

31 Yamazaki F, Hamasaki K. Heat acclimation increases skin vasodilation and sweating but not cardiac baroreflex responses in heat-stressed humans. *J Appl Physiol (1985)* 2003 Oct;95(4):1567–74.

32 Lorenzo S, Halliwill JR, Sawka MN, Minson CT. Heat acclimation improves exercise performance. *J Appl Physiol (1985)* 2010 Oct;109(4):1140–7.

33 Nielsen B, Hales JR, Strange S, Christensen NJ, Warberg J, Saltin B. Human circulatory and thermoregulatory adaptations with heat acclimation and exercise in a hot, dry environment. *J Physiol* 1993 Jan;460:467–85.

34 Nielsen B, Strange S, Christensen NJ, Warberg J, Saltin B. Acute and adaptive responses in humans to exercise in a warm, humid environment. *Pflugers Arch* 1997 May;434(1):49–56.

35 Wyndham CH, Benade AJ, Williams CG, Strydom NB, Goldin A, Heyns AJ. Changes in central circulation and body fluid spaces during acclimatization to heat. *J Appl Physiol* 1968 Nov;25(5):586–93.

36 Patterson MJ, Stocks JM, Taylor NA. Sustained and generalized extracellular fluid expansion following heat acclimation. *J Physiol* 2004 Aug 15;559(Pt 1):327–34.

37 Horvath SM, Shelley WB. Acclimatization to extreme heat and its effect on the ability to work in less severe environments. *Am J Physiol* 1946 Jun;146:336–43.

38 Lorenzo S, Minson CT. Heat acclimation improves cutaneous vascular function and sweating in trained cyclists. *J Appl Physiol (1985)* 2010 Dec;109(6):1736–43.

39 Armstrong CG, Kenney WL. Effects of age and acclimation on responses to passive heat exposure. *J Appl Physiol (1985)* 1993 Nov;75(5):2162–7.

40 Beaudin AE, Walsh ML, White MD. Central chemoreflex ventilatory responses in humans following passive heat acclimation. *Respir Physiol Neurobiol* 2012 Jan 15;180(1):97–104.

41 Henane R, Bittel J. Changes of thermal balance induced by passive heating in resting man. *J Appl Physiol* 1975 Feb;38(2):294–9.

42 Mitchell D, Senay LC, Wyndham CH, van Rensburg AJ, Rogers GG, Strydom NB. Acclimatization in a hot, humid environment: energy exchange, body temperature, and sweating. *J Appl Physiol* 1976 May;40(5):768–78.

43 Candas V, Libert JP, Vogt JJ. Effect of hidromeiosis on sweat drippage during acclimation to humid heat. *Eur J Appl Physiol Occup Physiol* 1980;44(2):123–33.

44 Ormerod JK, Elliott TA, Scheett TP, Vanheest JL, Armstrong LE, Maresh CM. Drinking behavior and perception of thirst in untrained women during 6 weeks of heat acclimation and outdoor training. *Int J Sport Nutr Exerc Metab* 2003 Mar;13(1):15–28.

45 Sunderland C, Morris JG, Nevill ME. A heat acclimation protocol for team sports. *Br J Sports Med* 2008 May;42(5):327–33.

46 Yeargin SW, Casa DJ, Armstrong LE, Watson G, Judelson DA, Psathas E, et al. Heat acclimatization and hydration status of American football players during initial summer workouts. *J Strength Cond Res* 2006 Aug;20(3):463–70.

47 Petersen CJ, Portus MR, Pyne DB, Dawson BT, Cramer MN, Kellett AD. Partial heat acclimation in cricketers using a 4-day high intensity cycling protocol. *Int J Sports Physiol Perform* 2010 Dec;5(4):535–45.

48 Magalhaes FC, Passos RL, Fonseca MA, Oliveira KP, Ferreira-Junior JB, Martini AR, et al. Thermoregulatory efficiency is increased after heat acclimation in tropical natives. *J Physiol Anthropol* 2010;29(1):1–12.

49 Neal RA, Corbett J, Massey HC, Tipton MJ. Effect of short-term heat acclimation with permissive dehydration on thermoregulation and temperate exercise performance. *Scand J Med Sci Sports* 2015 Jul 29.

50 Lee BJ, Miller A, James RS, Thake CD. Cross acclimation between heat and hypoxia: heat acclimation improves cellular tolerance and exercise performance in acute normobaric hypoxia. *Front Physiol* 2016;7:78.

51 Racinais S, Buchheit M, Bilsborough J, Bourdon PC, Cordy J, Coutts AJ. Physiological and performance responses to a training camp in the heat in professional Australian football players. *Int J Sports Physiol Perform* 2014 Jul;9(4):598–603.

52 de DR, Brager GS. The adaptive model of thermal comfort and energy conservation in the built environment. *Int J Biometeorol* 2001 Jul;45(2):100–8.

53 King DS, Costill DL, Fink WJ, Hargreaves M, Fielding RA. Muscle metabolism during exercise in the heat in unacclimatized and acclimatized humans. *J Appl Physiol (1985)* 1985 Nov;59(5):1350–4.

54 Magalhaes FC, Amorim FT, Passos RL, Fonseca MA, Oliveira KP, Lima MR, et al. Heat and exercise acclimation increases intracellular levels of Hsp72 and inhibits exercise-induced increase in intracellular and plasma Hsp72 in humans. *Cell Stress Chaperones* 2010 Nov;15(6):885–95.

55 Galloway SDR, Maughan RJ. Effects of ambient temperature on the capacity to perform prolonged exercise in man. *Med Sci Sports Exerc* 1997;29:1240–9.

56 Buchheit M, Voss SC, Nybo L, Mohr M, Racinais S. Physiological and performance adaptations to an in-season soccer camp in the heat: associations with heart rate and heart rate variability. *Scand J Med Sci Sports* 2011 Dec;21(6):e477–e485.

57 Buchheit M, Racinais S, Bilsborough J, Hocking J, Mendez-Villanueva A, Bourdon PC, et al. Adding heat to the live-high train-low altitude model: a practical insight from professional football. *Br J Sports Med* 2013 Dec;47 Suppl 1:i59–i69.

58 Shvartz E, Shapiro Y, Magazanik A, Meroz A, Birnfeld H, Mechtinger A, et al. Heat acclimation, physical fitness, and responses to exercise in temperate and hot environments. *J Appl Physiol Respir Environ Exerc Physiol* 1977 Oct;43(4):678–83.

59 White AC, Salgado RM, Astorino TA, Loeppky JA, Schneider SM, McCormick JJ, et al. The effect of 10 days of heat acclimation on exercise performance in acute hypobaric hypoxia (4350 m). *Temperature (Austin)* 2016 Jan;3(1):176–85.

60 Gibson OR, Turner G, Tuttle JA, Taylor L, Watt PW, Maxwell NS. Heat acclimation attenuates physiological strain and the HSP72, but not HSP90alpha, mRNA response to acute normobaric hypoxia. *J Appl Physiol (1985)* 2015 Oct 15;119(8):889–99.

61 Maloyan A, Eli-Berchoer L, Semenza GL, Gerstenblith G, Stern MD, Horowitz M. HIF-1alpha-targeted pathways are activated by heat acclimation and contribute to acclimation-ischemic cross-tolerance in the heart. *Physiol Genomics* 2005 Sep 21;23(1):79–88.

62 Daanen HAM, Racinais S, Periard JD. Heat acclimation decay and re-induction: a systematic review and meta-analysis. *Sports Med* 2018 Feb;48(2):409–30.

63 Ashley CD, Ferron J, Bernard TE. Loss of heat acclimation and time to re-establish acclimation. *J Occup Environ Hyg* 2015;12(5):302–8.

64 Garrett AT, Goosens NG, Rehrer NJ, Patterson MJ, Cotter JD. Induction and decay of short-term heat acclimation. *Eur J Appl Physiol* 2009 Dec;107(6):659–70.

65 Daanen HA, Jonkman AG, Layden JD, Linnane DM, Weller AS. Optimising the acquisition and retention of heat acclimation. *Int J Sports Med* 2011 Nov;32(11):822–8.

66 Pichan G, Sridharan K, Swamy YV, Joseph S, Gautam RK. Physiological acclimatization to heat after a spell of cold conditioning in tropical subjects. *Aviat Space Environ Med* 1985 May;56(5):436–40.

67 Stephens RL, Hoag LL. Heat acclimatization, its decay and reinduction in young Caucasian females. *Am Ind Hyg Assoc J* 1981 Jan;42(1):12–7.

68 Saat M, Sirisinghe RG, Singh R, Tochihara Y. Decay of heat acclimation during exercise in cold and exposure to cold environment. *Eur J Appl Physiol* 2005 Oct;95(4):313–20.

69 Williams CG, Wyndham CH, Morrison JF. Rate of loss of acclimatization in summer and winter. *J Appl Physiol* 1967 Jan;22(1):21–6.

70 Pandolf KB, Burse RL, Goldman RF. Role of physical fitness in heat acclimatisation, decay and reinduction. *Ergonomics* 1977 Jul;20(4):399–408.

71 Lind AR, Bass DE. Optimal exposure time for development of acclimatization to heat. *Fed Proc* 1963 May;22:704–8.

72 Weller AS, Linnane DM, Jonkman AG, Daanen HA. Quantification of the decay and re-induction of heat acclimation in dry-heat following 12 and 26 days without exposure to heat stress. *Eur J Appl Physiol* 2007 Dec;102(1):57–66.

7

COOLING

What should you know by the end of the chapter?

As discussed in the previous chapter, heat acclimation can be a highly effective strategy to combat the negative effect of high internal and external temperatures on exercise performance; however, it is not always practical, as it requires time and resources (e.g. the ability to travel to a warm country or access to an environmental chamber). Alternative strategies that can alleviate the impaired performance are required for situations where time and/or resources are limited and cooling the body (or parts of the body) is one such strategy. Depending on the demands and restrictions of the sport, athletes can be cooled before, during, and/or after exercise using both internal and external approaches. By the end of this chapter you should know the following:

- How and when athlete cooling strategies can be used
- The effect of different cooling approaches on exercise performance
- The effect of different cooling approaches on the physiological and perceptual response to exercise

Key terms for this chapter

After-drop	A delayed reduction in core body temperature often observed following cold-water immersion. This occurs because cold-water immersion can result in vasoconstriction and the cooled peripheral blood can only circulate once vasodilation occurs.
Cold-water immersion	The immersion of the body (whole or partial) in cold or cool water.

Effect size	Effect sizes quantify the difference between groups and are sometimes used in place of significance testing. The larger the effect size, the larger the difference. Cohen's *d* and Hedges' *g* effect sizes are reported in this chapter. Hedges' *g* is better for small studies (<20 participants) because it is more conservative.
External cooling	Cooling the outside surface of the body
Ice vests	A cooling garment designed to cool the torso. *Ice vest, cooling vest, ice jacket,* and *cooling jacket* are terms that are used somewhat interchangeably in the literature.
Internal cooling	Cooling the body from within e.g. by ingesting cold/iced fluids.
Per-cooling	Cooling administered during exercise/periods of activity.
Pre-cooling	Cooling administered before exercise/periods of activity.

Problem 7.1: Cooling an elite time-trial cyclist

You are the physiologist for the Olympic cycling team, who have a 54.5 km time trial in 24 h time. A sudden heat wave means that there is a spike in temperature. What cooling strategies would you recommend and why? How and when should they be used?

7.1 Cooling in elite sport

Despite regular media stories reporting athletes cooling themselves before and during exercise and photos of athletes either immersed in cold water, drinking cold drinks, or wearing a range of cooling garments (homemade or shop-bought!), actual data regarding the use of cooling strategies in elite sport are scarce.

Quick question: Table 7.1 lists the cooling strategies most commonly used. Before reading on, have a think about what advantages and disadvantages each has and when they might be used by athletes. By the end of this chapter, the table will be complete!

The 2015 IAAF World Championships in Beijing were expected to be hot and were hot (mean wet-bulb global temperature = 24–27°C at midday and 25–30°C at 4pm) and so Julien Périard and colleagues (1) asked athletes what cooling strategies they planned to use. Three hundred and seven athletes responded and just over half (52%) of those planned to use at least one cooling strategy during the Championships. Figure 7.1 shows the range of strategies planned for by athletes from a variety of events.

Unsurprisingly, athletes who reported having previously suffered an exertional heat illness were more likely to adopt a cooling strategy, so were athletes from Africa and Asia (compared to those from Australia, North America, or South America), female athletes (58% versus 48% of males), and those competing in endurance events (1). Endurance athletes are more likely to adopt cooling

TABLE 7.1 Table summarising the most commonly used cooling strategies

Cooling approach	Internal?	External?	Pre-cooling?	Per-cooling?	Pros	Cons
Whole-body cold water immersion						
Lower-body cold water immersion						
Ice vest						
Cooling collar/hood						
Fans and water spray						
Ice/cold-water ingestion						
Menthol						

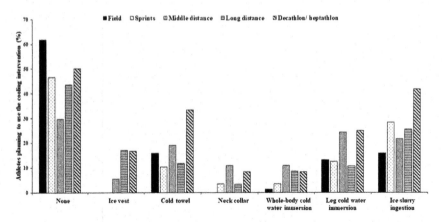

FIGURE 7.1 The percentage of athletes who reported planning to use a specific cooling strategy during the 2015 IAAF World Championships in Beijing. Figure drawn from data extracted from Périard et al. (1).

interventions due to the greater exposure times and thermal strain that they will experience in completion and training; however, the reasons for the other differences are not clear.

7.2 When to cool?

Cooling can be applied before, during, and/or after exercise. Cooling before exercising is known as pre-cooling ("pre" means "before" in Latin) whereas cooling during exercise is called per-cooling (from the Latin for "through"). Pre- and per-cooling in isolation and in combination will be discussed here. Post-exercise cooling is often used as part of a recovery regimen and/or to cool hyperthermic athletes – the latter will be discussed in Chapter 9.

7.2.1 Cooling before exercise

The aim of pre-cooling is to enable the athlete to start the exercise bout with a lower level of physiological and perceptual strain to enable them to either exercise for longer or to exercise harder e.g. adopt a faster pace. Many athletes cool prior to competing or training in the heat and do so using a variety of methods such as cold-water immersion, cooling garments, or cold/iced fluid ingestion. Pre-cooling can affect subsequent exercise performance in a number of ways ranging from small impairment to very large improvement (Figure 7.2) and the differences are usually due to differences in the magnitude of cooling offered, the thermal strain experienced, the thermal stress faced, the exercise duration, or a combination of these. Bogerd et al. (2) conducted a meta-analysis (a type of systematic review) which suggested that combining a variety of pre-cooling approaches ("Mixed-method" cooling) may be optimal (Figure 7.3). Cohen's

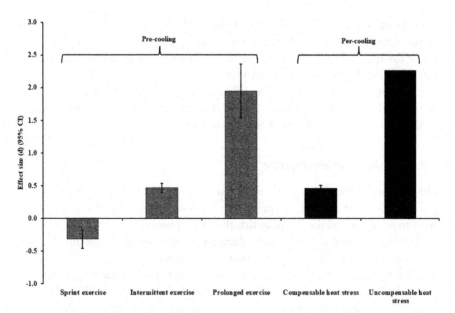

FIGURE 7.2 Effect sizes observed with pre- and per-cooling approaches broken down by activity (for pre-cooling) and heat stress (for per-cooling). Data extracted from the meta-analysis conducted by Tyler et al. (3).

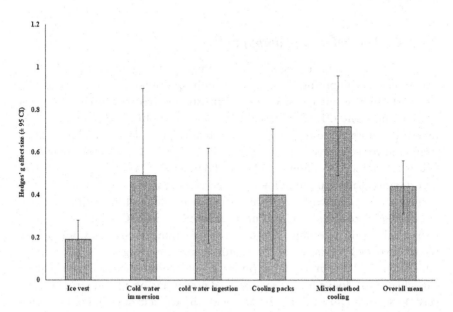

FIGURE 7.3 The effect size (Hedges' g ± 95% confidence intervals) of different pre-cooling approaches. Drawn from data presented by Bongers et al. (21).

d and Hedges' *g* are effect sizes that can be used to measure by how much two groups differ from one another and overall effect sizes can be calculated regardless of the original unit of measurement (e.g. studies reporting changes in time and power can be combined). The larger the effect size, the larger the difference so we can see in Figure 7.3 that the difference in performance with and without mixed-method cooling (Hedges' *g* = 0.72) is 3.8 times greater than the difference observed with and without an ice vest (Hedges' *g* = 0.19).

7.2.2 Cooling during exercise

The benefits of pre-cooling are often lost or diminished during exercise (4–9) and so cooling during exercise (per-cooling) has been investigated and utilised in order to try to extend the duration that the participants experience a lower actual or perceived thermal strain. Cooling during exercise is an appealing intervention but a number of practical considerations may restrict or prevent its use e.g. the laws and regulations of the sport, excess weight, and skin irritation (4). A number of per-cooling interventions have been tested and these include cold air exposure (10), torso cooling using an ice vest (4;11–13), neck cooling using a cooling collar (14–17), and cold beverage/ice slurry ingestion (18;19). Per-cooling is sometimes, somewhat confusingly, also called mid-cooling (20) but to avoid confusion with half-time (mid-event) cooling interventions, (which are a combination of pre- (before the second half) and post- (after the first half) cooling) per-cooling is more appropriate.

7.2.3 Cooling before and during exercise

Pre- and per-cooling strategies can be combined to try to harness the benefits of each. Combining pre- and per-cooling strategies can improve exercise performance but the size of the benefits reported is similar to pre- or per-cooling alone (21;22). Internal pre- and per-cooling ingesting cold fluid ingestion before and during exercise can reduce physiological and perceptual strain and improve cycling capacity in the heat by ~23% (23) but beneficial effects are not always observed (24;25). Riera et al. (24) and Tran et al. (25) reported no change in physiological or perceptual strain and only observed a performance benefit with ice slushy (rather than cold fluid) ingestion, whereas Lee et al. (23) reported 4°C was more effective than 37°C fluid. Pre-cooling individuals using a combination of ice slurry (internal pre-cooling) and ice towels (external pre-cooling) for 30 min prior to cycling in the heat during which time ad libitum ice slurry (internal), per-cooling was allowed enabled participants to adopt a higher self-selected power during a fixed rating of perceived exertion (RPE) test (19). Although the participants adopted a higher power output, the combined approach was no better than the per-cooling intervention alone.

7.3 Cooling methods

Athletes use a variety of cooling methods before and during exercise which can be applied either externally or internally. External cooling interventions attempt to reduce the actual and perceived levels of thermal strain experienced by directly cooling the skin, peripheral blood, and superficial tissues, whereas internal cooling directly cools the tissues from the oral cavity to the stomach. External and internal approaches can also be combined. As mentioned, the effectiveness of a cooling intervention used depends on a number of factors such as the magnitude of cooling provided, the thermal strain experienced, and the exercise intensity, whereas the practicality depends on the specific nature of the sport and the window of opportunity available to cool.

This section will help with Problem 7.1: Cooling an elite time-trial cyclist: "You are the physiologist for the Olympic cycling team who have a 54.5 km time-trial in 24 h time. A sudden heat wave means that there is a spike in temperature. What cooling strategies would you recommend and why? How and when should they be used?"

Make sure that you consider the information about when to apply cooling covered in the previous section.

Quick question: Before we move on, what cooling strategies have you seen athletes use (perhaps on television)? Think about what sport you saw that cooling approach used in, would it work in different sports? Would it be legal or practical?

7.3.1 Cold-water immersion

Cold-water immersion involves the immersion of the body (whole or partial) in cold or cool water (usually 2–26°C). Whole-body cold-water immersion is the most effective way of cooling the body but it lacks practicality, which may explain why more athletes planned to use lower limb cold-water immersion, than whole-body cold-water immersion, at the 2015 IAAF World Championships in Beijing (1). A number of studies have looked at cooling sections of the body using water immersion and these have included cooling non-active (e.g. torso (26) or hands (27)) and active (e.g. legs (28)) body parts.

Cold-water immersion can be used as part of a pre-cooling or post-cooling regimen (and per-cooling during activities such as swimming and surfing). Cold-water immersion can directly remove heat from the body by cooling the peripheral tissues and blood. The cooled blood then circulates to the central regions of the body cooling them as it does. Immersion of the body in cold water leads to peripheral vasoconstriction, which reduces the peripheral blood volume and shifts the blood centrally. This redistribution of blood increases the central blood volume and can subsequently increase stroke volume allowing for a lower heart rate at a given exercise intensity (5;29;30). If the water is too cold, peripheral vasoconstriction may be too severe and could shut off peripheral blood flow entirely. If this happens, heat can no longer be lost, and the uncooled blood moves centrally raising core body temperature. Once the athlete is removed from the cold water, peripheral blood flow can be restored and the cold peripheral blood can once again circulate to the core. This causes a delayed reduction in core body temperature termed an *after-drop*. The lower skin temperatures observed during cold-water immersion change the perceived thermal state and thermal comfort of the athlete (5;31;32). Whether the reduction in skin temperature is perceived as pleasant or unpleasant depends on the magnitude of cooling presented. The colder the water, the more unpleasant the sensations are likely to be (33), especially when large surface areas are immersed (34).

As shown in Figure 7.3, pre-cooling using cold-water immersion has an overall benefit effect on subsequent exercise but the response is far from consistent (note the large confidence intervals). It is often said that lowering the temperature of the muscles required by the sport should be avoided because reductions in muscle temperature can extend the time-to-peak tension, decrease voluntary power output (35), and slow the rate of anaerobic metabolism (31;36); however, improvements in short-duration (<15 min) exercise have been observed. Figure 7.2 highlights that the benefit of pre-cooling is related to the exercise type being undertaken and that sprint exercise is usually impaired. Muscle temperature was not measured in the studies conducted by Marsh and Sleivert (26) or Yeargin et al. (37) that were included in the meta-analysis that yielded the data in Figure 7.2 but it is likely that muscle temperature was lower following cold-water immersion because Castle et al. (38) observed a reduction in muscle temperature of ~1.5°C following cold-water immersion. Castle et al. (38) reported that cold-water immersion did not improve the work done during an intermittent cycling sprint test but cold-water immersion pre-cooling appears to benefit prolonged, continuous exercise. Cold-water immersion prior to prolonged (30–63 min) exercise consistently improves subsequent exercise performance and capacity (+4–37%) (5;6;8;29). In one such investigation, Gonzalez-Alonso et al. (29) pre-cooled participants by ~1.5°C using cold-water immersion. The rate of heat storage and the core temperature at volitional exercise termination were identical to control group (+0.8°C), but pre-cooling extended the time taken to reach exhaustion by 17 min.

7.3.2 Ice vests

Practical torso cooling has been somewhat commonplace in elite sport since the mid-1990s when the Australian Institute of Sport began piloting their use with members of the Australian National road cycling squad (39). *Ice vest*, *cooling vest*, *ice jacket*, and *cooling jacket* are terms that are used interchangeably in the literature to describe these cooling garments, but *ice vest* is the most commonly used name and so will be used here. Ice vests can contain cooling sections that contain phase-change materials that are activated by water and cooled in

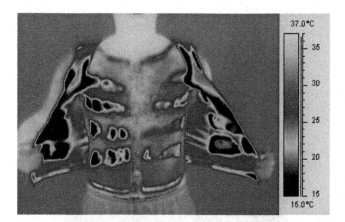

FIGURE 7.4 Thermal image showing the localised cooling offered by an Arctic Heat cooling vest – note that you can see where is (darker patches), and where isn't (lighter patches), being cooled.

refrigerators, freezers, or iced water, or make use of frozen or cooled liquid (usually water) inserts. Vests typically cover the entire torso (~25% of the body surface area (12)); however, the actual surface area cooled is often much less (5–10% (12;13)) due to the design of the vests and location of the cooling strips/packs (Figure 7.4). Ice vests are worn either directly on the skin or over the top of a thin clothing layer (sometimes a wet layer to aid cooling) to facilitate conductive and evaporative cooling.

Ice vests (an example is pictured in Figure 7.5) can be worn before, during, or after exercise but are most frequently used before exercise, during active warm-ups, or during periods of rest e.g. substitutes may wear them while on the bench prior to coming on. Commercially available cooling vests weigh between 0.5 and 4.5 kg (4;40) with the most commonly investigated one (Arctic Heat) weighing ~1.5 kg when activated (2). The energy cost of movement increases when carrying a load (41), and so wearing a cooling garment during exercise is likely to increase the energy demands. There is no additional energy cost of wearing an ice vest during cycling (13) but the impact on the energy cost of load-bearing activities such as running is unknown. Arngrimsson et al. (4) investigated one of the heaviest vests (4.5 kg) and reduced the warm-up running speed by ~0.8 km·h^{-1} *"to compensate for the extra metabolic work done... due to the weight of the vest"* (p. 1868).

When worn as part of a pre-cooling routine, ice vests can lower core body temperature, skin temperature, and heart rate (4;42–44) but not all ice vests offer a sufficiently cooling effect to induce prolonged reductions (3;22). For example, Castle et al. (38) pre-cooled participants for 20 min using an ice vest prior to a 40 min intermittent sprint protocol and although rectal temperature was reduced throughout, heart rate was unaffected, and skin temperature was reduced for only about 8 min. Similarly, Arngrimsson et al. (4) reported that

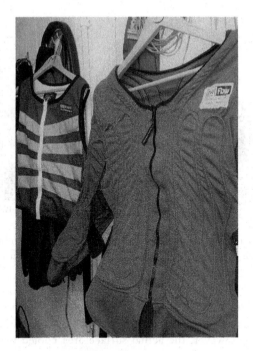

FIGURE 7.5 An ice vest and liquid-cooled cooling jacket.

wearing an ice vest during an active warm-up reduced core and skin tempera-ture, and lowered heart rate but that the reductions had disappeared before the end of the 5 km time trial. Per-cooling using vests can reduce physiological strain but may only do so when the magnitude of heat stress is very high (11). Kenny et al. (11) reported that wearing an ice vest under a nuclear, biological, and chemical protective clothing reduced core and skin temperatures during walking but other studies have reported that in less thermally challenging set-tings, per-cooling the torso had no effect on rectal temperature, mean skin temperature, or heart rate (12;13). Ice vest pre-cooling can improve the per-ception of task difficulty and thermal comfort (4;42–44); however, not all vests offer a sufficiently prolonged cooling effect to induce such changes (3;22). Ice vests worn during exercise can improve thermal sensations (12;13) and so com-bining pre- and per-cooling approaches may be effective. Unless the magnitude of heat strain is very high, it appears that any benefits that arise due to wearing occur because of the sum effect of small beneficial physiological changes and reductions in perceived physiological strain (12;13) rather than large individual changes in any single variable.

Figure 7.3 shows that on average there is a small benefit of wearing an ice vest but the confidence intervals suggest that the benefit is far from consistently observed. Arngrimsson et al. (4) reported that pre-cooling using an ice vest worn during an active warm-up improved subsequent 5 km time-trial performance by 1.1% and the majority of studies report benefits of similar magnitude or slightly larger (1–14%). Per-cooling with an ice vest can improve exercise capacity by ~12% when worn under nuclear, biological, and chemical protective clothing (11) (see Figure 7.2) and by 17–21% in less thermally challenging settings (12;13).

7.3.3 Head and neck cooling garments

There are some practical issues with torso cooling (e.g. the need to remove clothing, the mass of the vest, ease of availability) and so some athletes make use of head and neck cooling devices. Despite only making up ~1% (13) and ~8% (65) of the body surface area, respectively, it is not uncommon to see tennis players cooling the neck and head with home-made ice towels during warm weather tournaments and more recently the use of commercially available devices has been observed in sports such as Formula 1.

Ice vests and neck cooling collars can be worn before, during, or after exercise. Research has investigated pre- and per-cooling but in sporting events head and neck cooling garments are most frequently used during active warm-ups or periods of rest e.g. between games in tennis. Cooling the head and neck regions rarely has any effect on physiological strain with most studies reporting no changes in physiological, hormonal, or biochemical variables (12;14–17;45–48). Reductions in thermal and cardiovascular strain have been reported but only when the entire head is cooled and the participant is under severe thermal strain (49). Head and neck cooling does not reduce core body temperature during exercise when measured rectally, but some have suggested that it may lower brain temperature. The main determinant of brain temperature is the temperature of the blood in the internal carotid artery (50) and Cabanac (51) proposed that countercurrent heat exchange between the superficial arteries and veins in the neck region might lower brain temperature by removing heat on route to the brain. This idea is based upon selective brain cooling – an evolutionary advantage that frequently preyed-upon animals have to allow them to tolerate very high core body temperatures, while maintaining lower brain temperatures, to allow them to escape a predator. These species are able to lower the temperature of the blood on route to the brain by utilising countercurrent heat exchange between arterial and venous blood. Selective brain cooling appears unlikely to occur in humans because the high cerebral blood flow velocity in humans limits the opportunity for heat exchange (52;53) and there is an insufficient temperature difference between the arterial and venous blood (52). Externally cooling the head and neck regions could conceivably lower the temperature of the carotid blood destined for the brain and thus lower the temperature of the brain (54); however, the deep brain temperature is practically homogenous (55) and external cooling is unlikely to alter this (56;57). Although unlikely to reduce physiological strain, the neck and head have high levels of alliesthesial thermosensitivity (58) and may provide a greater thermoregulatory advantage compared to cooling other parts of the body (49;59–61) and elicit disproportionately beneficial changes in perceived thermal strain (62). Cooling the body at any site can alter the perception of thermal comfort and sensation and this is the case when cooling the neck; however, the benefits of cooling on thermal comfort (46;59;60;63–70) are not always matched with alterations in the participants' perception of the task difficulty as expressed via the RPE scale (16;46;47;69;70). Per-cooling the head and neck regions can improve running performance (~6%) and capacity (~13%) in hot environments (17;80;96–99) resulting in a mean improvement of 7%; however, the improvements are not always statistically significant (+6% (17); +9% (80)). Pre-cooling data are lacking despite the aforementioned use in the field (e.g. tennis and motorsport).

7.3.4 Fan cooling

Quick question: We covered the effects of wind speed on thermal stress and strain in Chapter 3. Based on what you know, why might fan cooling be beneficial to an athlete?

Fan cooling mimics the convective heat loss experienced naturally when exercising with an airflow e.g. a natural breeze or the airflow created as you cycle. Fan cooling aims to remove the warm air that occupies the space immediately above the skin's surface to widen the air–skin temperature gradient and facilitate heat loss. Ecologically valid airflow is often missing in exercise physiology research conducted in environmental conditions (71) and the lack of a representative airflow means that the effects of other heat-mitigating interventions (e.g. cooling) might be overstated (72;73). While many sports naturally generate an airflow (e.g. cycling), the opportunities to use artificial airflow in elite sport are limited predominantly to periods of seated rest e.g. whilst on the substitutes bench or at the change of ends in tennis.

Convective and evaporative heat loss is increased proportionally as airflow increases (74), and so it is unsurprising that fan cooling can lower core body temperature, skin temperature, sweat rate, and heart rate (74–78). The reductions in physiological strain are often matched with RPE and thermal sensation (72;74;77;78). Fan cooling is often used in combination with skin wetting to further increase evaporative heat loss and Lynch et al. (79) highlighted the added benefit of doing so. Fan cooling with water spray effectively lowered physiological strain in a tennis simulation study (77) but without a fan-only condition, it was unclear to what extent the fan and/or water spray explained the reduction. Lynch et al. (79) undertook another tennis simulation study but this time directly compared fan cooling only with fan cooling administered alongside a water spray. Fan cooling with the water spray resulted in lower rectal temperatures, skin temperatures, heart rate, sweat rates, and perceived exertion and thermal sensation compared to fan cooling without the water spray (79).

Fan cooling may impair short-duration cycling capacity (369 s versus 399 s) (67) but appears to consistently improve prolonged exercise performance and capacity. Otani et al. (74) compared the effects of 0, 10, 20, or 30 km·h^{-1}

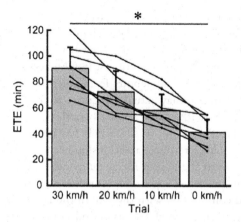

FIGURE 7.6 Progressive reduction in exercise capacity observed in the heat as airspeed was reduced in the study by Otani et al. (74). Applied physiology, nutrition, and metabolism by Canadian Science Publishing. Reproduced with permission of Canadian Science Publishing in the format Republish in a book via Copyright Clearance Center.

airspeeds on cycling to exhaustion in hot conditions. Exercise capacity time was progressively shortened as airspeed reduced with a reduction of ~16 min for every 10 $km·h^{-1}$ decrease in airflow (Figure 7.6). The greatest capacity was observed with the greatest airspeed (30 $km·h^{-1}$; 90.3 ± 16.5 min) and this was ~50 min longer than the cycling capacity observed with no airflow at all (41.4 ± 10.1 min). Similar improvements were reported by Ansley et al. (10) who observed that head and face fan and water spray cooling increased cycling capacity in the heat by ~51% (median average). As well as improving open-loop capacity test performance, fan cooling can improve exercise performance and recently it was reported that fan cooling increased the exercise time during a tennis simulation in the heat (77) compared to the currently adopted ice-towel approach and no cooling.

7.3.5 Menthol cooling

Menthol cooling is a cooling method that involves the application of menthol to either the skin (usually as a gel or spray) or the oral cavity (as a mouth rinse or ingested with a cold or ice-slush beverage (24;25;80–82). Menthol is an alcohol produced either naturally from mint oils or synthetically and can be found in a number of forms although L-menthol is the most common. Menthol was not mentioned in the athlete survey conducted by Périard et al. (1) and so it is not known how widely used it is; however, due to its ease and range of application, menthol could be applied before, during, or after exercise. Menthol can cause irritation to the eyes and nose, so this should be considered.

Menthol does not reduce physiological strain (83–86) but activates the same receptors (transient receptor potential ion channel Melastatin 8 (TRPM8 for short)) activated by air temperatures between 8°C and 28°C (87;88) to give the sensation of cooling during bouts of rest (89;90) and exercise (91;92). This means that menthol can make somebody feel cooler but it will not reduce actual physiological stain and may actually increase it (91;93). Menthol concentrations between 1% and 10% cause vasoconstriction, reduce skin blood flow, and delay the onset of sweating in some (94) but not all (95;96) studies and there appears to be a dose–response relationship between the concentration of menthol and the rate in the rise of rectal temperature (94;97). In contrast to physiological strain, menthol application consistently improves the perceived thermal strain and comfort. As with the rate in the rise of rectal temperature, the impact of perceived thermal sensation and comfort appears to be dose-dependent with participants reporting a greater cooling sensation with a 0.2% menthol spray compared to a 0.05% one (91) although lower strengths can improve perceived thermal strain when mouth rinsed (0.01%) or ingested (0.05%) (24;25;80–82).

Quick question: Why do many mouthwashes, toothpastes, and "freeze sprays" feel cool? Take a look at yours and see whether they contain menthol.

Despite mainly only improving perceived rather than actual strain, menthol can improve exercise performance and capacity in the heat. Applying menthol gel (8%) to the face can increase the work completed at a fixed RPE by 21% (86) but weaker external applications (0.05% menthol sprayed on to clothing) do not improve exercise performance (83–85). Similar and weaker menthol concentrations can be effective at improving exercise performance if rinsed in the mouth (0.01%) or ingested (0.05%) (24;25;80–82) suggesting that there may be a greater sensitivity to menthol/cold here.

7.3.6 Cold beverage ingestion

In addition to menthol ingestion or mouth rinsing, internal cooling can be achieved by ingesting or mouth rinsing with cold or iced beverages. As long as the drinks can be kept, or made, cold/iced, cold beverage ingestion can take place any time that fluids can be consumed – before, during, and after exercise (see Chapter 8 for more of hydration) – although some restrictions will exist based on sports regulations (i.e. are drinks breaks permitted?) and athlete tolerance issues (e.g. can your athlete drink sufficient cold/iced beverages without experiencing gastrointestinal issues?).

Drinking a cold or iced beverage can directly cool the tissues that the fluid comes into contact with (e.g. the mouth) but can also lower starting core temperature and slow the rate at which it rises during exercise in the heat (7;18;23). Drinking an ice slurry can approximately double the heat sink, compared to that created by drinking a cold beverage because of the combined thermodynamic properties of ice (specific heat capacity = 2.1 $kJ \cdot kg^{-1} \cdot {}^{\circ}C^{-1}$) and liquid water (specific heat capacity $= 4.2 \text{ kJ} \cdot \text{kg}^{-1} \cdot {}^\circ\text{C}^{-1}$). Due to the greater heat sink, it is unsurprising that ice slurry ingestion before and during exercise can reduce core body temperature (30;98–101); however, reductions are not always observed (102). Internal per-cooling does not consistently reduce core body temperature (18;19;103–105) and recent data have recommended that ice slurries should not be ingested during exercise in the heat – especially by novice athletes who are more susceptible to heat illness (105). This is because cooling from within can suppress the sudomotor response to heat, reducing sweat rate, sweat loss, and evaporative heat loss from the skin (23;30;100;103–106) and subsequently increasing heat storage during exercise in the heat (100;105). If observed, the magnitude of re-duction in core body temperature is strongly related to the temperature of the in-gested fluid with greater reductions observed with the ingestion of colder drinks (106). As mentioned in Chapter 2, gut permeability increases as core body tem-perature increases and so it has been proposed that direct internal cooling might preserve gut integrity. Limited data exist but Snipe and Costa (101) reported that ingesting cool (7°C) or cold (0°C) fluid before and during exertional heat stress only slightly decreases gastrointestinal injury and upper gastrointestinal symptoms and does not affect systemic inflammatory cytokines in well-trained euhydrated endurance athletes (101).

While thermoreceptors in or around the stomach appear to be responsible for alterations in sweating (105;107), the stimulation of thermal receptors in both the oral and abdominal regions can improve perceived thermal strain despite poten-tial increases in heat strain (108). Interestingly, internal cooling may have a dis-proportionate effect on improving perceived thermal strain as demonstrated by Siegel et al. (30) who reported that despite cold-water immersion reducing core body temperature to a greater extent than ice slurry ingestion alone, combining the ice slurry and cold-water immersion had no additive benefit and improved thermal sensation to a similar extent (30). Data regarding the effect of internal per-cooling on exercise performance are limited but positive. Cold (4°C) fluid and ice slurry ingestion can improve cycling capacity (by 13%) (18) and per-formance (by ~ 2.5% (19)) by allowing athletes to adopt a higher self-selected exercise intensity in the heat. A faster cycling or running speed would be advan-tageous if done within safe limits.

7.3.7 Mixed-method cooling

In an attempt to maximise the benefit of the different cooling interventions, sometimes the various approaches are combined. The combination of two or more individual cooling approaches has been called "mixed-method cool-ing" (2). A recent meta-analysis by Bogerd et al. (2) reported that mixed-method pre-cooling was a more effective cooling approach for improving exercise per-formance (+7.3%) than cold-water immersion (+6.5%), cold-water/ice ingestion (+6.3%), cooling packs (+4.3%), or ice vests (+3.4%); however, Figure 7.3 high-lights a range of responses. Sleivert et al. (31) compared ice vest-only cooling with a mixed-method approach of ice vest and ice packs placed on the thigh. They reported that both cooling approaches reduced physiological strain, but that the ice vest cooling had no effect on 45 s sprint performance (−2%; Cohen's $d = -0.1$) and that the ice vest and packs impaired performance (−7%; Cohen's $d = -0.6$). Cotter et al. (109) used a similar approach, pre-cooling with an ice vest and cold air, and in one trial only with the addition of ice packs to the thigh. The ice vest and cold air reduced skin temperature, mean body temperature, and rectal temperature but the reductions were greater when the thigh was also cooled. Heart rate was reduced to a similar extent with each cooling approach. In contrast to Sleivert et al. (31), self-paced exercise performance was improved with the mixed-method cooling – by 15% with the ice packs and by 17% without. The differing data are likely to be due to the longer exercise test (15 min) and the greater endogenous heat produced during this time elevated muscle temperature.

Recent work investigating the use of ice packs, ice towels, and ice vests in cricketers has shown that although such an approach is not always successful in improving performance despite reducing physiological and perceptual strain (110), it can be. Minett et al. (111) reported that although 10 min of mixed cooling (the same combination as before) reduced physiological and perceptual strain, it had no effect on exercise performance. In contrast, 20 min of the same mixed-method cooling improved exercise performance by ~5% and had a greater effect on reducing physiological and perceptual strain than the shorter mixed-method cooling. These data suggest that just as there is a dose–response relationship between the volume of cooling and performance gains (112), there is also such a relationship between the duration of cooling and performance benefits (111).

7.4 The effect of cooling on cognitive performance in the heat

Thermal stress and strain can impair cognitive function (see Chapter 5), but data regarding the effect of cooling before or during exercise on cognitive performance are limited and mixed. Cooling the head and neck regions while at rest in a hot environment improves (113;114) or has no effect on attention (113;115;116) and improves (113) or has no effect (113;114;116) on memory. Early data reported that cooling the head improved reaction time and accuracy during investigations designed to simulate flying conditions (117) and more recently Gaoua et al. (113) reported that head cooling can partially reverse the hyperthermia-induced impairment in sustained visual attention and short-term memory capacity (113). In contrast, Simmons and colleagues (68) reported that cooling the head and neck regions had no effect on a 15 min battery of cognitive tests (simple reaction time, digit vigilance, choice reaction time, and rapid visual information processing). In the study by Gaoua et al. (113), despite improving some aspect of cognitive function, cooling the head had no effect on other measures of attention or on long-term memory capacity. The authors suggested that the differences may be due to the fact that short-term and long-term memory involve two differing regions of the brain (the frontal and temporal, respectively). Simmons et al. (68) did not cool the frontal area, and so these data in combination tentatively suggest that direct frontal cooling of the brain (forehead cooling) may be required (113;116) to improve such aspects of cognitive performance.

Problem 7.1 revisited: Cooling an elite time-trial cyclist

You are the physiologist for the Olympic cycling team who have a 54.5 km time trial in 24 h time. A sudden heat wave means that there is a spike in temperature. What cooling strategies would you recommend and why? How and when should they be used?

A sudden change in the weather can compromise an athlete's ability to perform but as discussed cooling can help minimise any impairment in performance. A sudden spike in temperature suggests that your athletes are unaccustomed to the heat and so would likely benefit from a cooling intervention that lowers both physiological and perceptual strain and with 24 h to prepare you can adopt both pre- and per-cooling strategies.

Pre-cooling

Pre-cooling approaches should be combined (2) and so the approach adopted should make use of a number of approaches. Cold-water immersion, ice vests, head and neck cooling devices, fans, and cold fluid ingestion could all be used at different periods of time prior to the race in an attempt to prolong the reduction in physiological and perceived thermal strain.

* Whole-body cold-water immersion is the most effective way of cooling the body and can be relatively easily done by using any container large enough for your athletes – you can buy specialist cold-water immersion pools, but it is not uncommon to see athletes immersed in paddling pools, bath tubs, and even wheelie-bins! Whatever you immerse your athlete in needs to be big enough to contain your athlete and water, and needs to be something that your athlete can get safely in and out of. Lowering the temperature of the muscles required by the sport should be avoided because doing so can decrease voluntary power output (35) (among other things) and so you may wish to avoid whole-body pre-cooling and pre-cool non-active muscle groups (e.g. torso (26)). Whole-body cold-water immersion prior to prolonged (30–63 min) exercise improves subsequent exercise performance and capacity (6;8;5;29); however, many of these studies have used exercise intensities below those expected in an elite, competitive 40 km cycling time trial.
* Using an ice vest is less effective than using whole-body water immersion, but it may be more practical to use this approach; elite cycling teams are

often seen per-cooling during a warm-up on a stationary bicycle, and ice vests can lower core body and skin temperatures, and heart rate (4;42–44). Not all ice vests offer a sufficiently cooling effect to induce prolonged reductions (3;22) and so the benefit might be short-lived. You could combine cold-water immersion and ice vests, i.e. get your athlete to wear an ice vest during an active warm-up following a period of cold-water immersion.

- Head and neck cooling devices can be worn prior to exercise although doing so is unlikely to reduce physiological strain (12;14–17;45–48). Cooling the head and neck regions can improve thermal comfort (119), and so this strategy could be used in combination with a more effective strategy e.g. in combination with the ice vest during the warm-up.

- Fan cooling during stationary bike warm-ups can mimic the cooling provided while cycling. Fan cooling can reduce physiological (74–78) and perceptual (72;74;77;78) strain, and is easy to do if electric power is available. If used, further increase the evaporative heat loss by wetting the skin (e.g. mist spraying) (79).

- Ice slurry ingestion can reduce core body temperature (30;98–101), but it does not always do so (102). Although the effects on lowering physiological strain may not always be observed, ice slurry ingestion may be as effective as cold-water immersion at improving perceived thermal strain (30).

Per-cooling

The demands of the event are such that you do not have many per-cooling options but the effects of pre-cooling are likely to wear off during the ~75 min race and so considering the use of cooling is advisable.

- Your athlete is likely to benefit from some convective cooling while they cycle. You could increase the heat loss potential of the airflow by making sure that your athlete's skin and clothing are wet (79) but care should be taken to ensure that doing so does not impede movement or lead to detrimental discomfort.

- Menthol does not reduce physiological strain (83–86) but can lower perceived strain (24;25;80–82). Using menthol as part of a locally applied gel or ingested solution could be an attractive approach but care must be taken to avoid irritation.

- Ingesting cold beverages can improve cycling performance (19), and so if competing with a water bottle, it would be advisable to ensure that the fluid contained is chilled (although keep an eye on the volume as volume = mass).

Using cooling garments is an option; however, ice vests and head/neck cooling devices are often cumbersome and are very likely to disrupt the athlete's performance by disturbing the aerodynamic set-up. This is especially the case for head and neck cooling devices because the cyclists will be wearing a safety helmet, but you could advise your athlete to pour cool water over their head to take advantage of improvements in thermal comfort by cooling this region.

An important thing to consider in this situation is that your athletes may not have any experience of the proposed cooling interventions, and so although those outlined may form an optimal strategy on paper, you would need to weigh up the benefits offered by the cooling interventions against any disruption or unrest caused by changes in the athletes' pre-race preparation routines.

7.5 Summary

Although data are limited, it is clear that elite athletes use a range of cooling interventions depending on the demands of their sport. Cooling can be applied before (pre-cooling) and/or during (per-cooling) depending on how practical it is to cool at that time and what the objectives of the cooling intervention are and athletes can be cooled using external and internal approaches. External cooling interventions attempt to reduce thermal strain experienced by directly cooling the skin, whereas internal cooling directly cools the tissues from the oral cavity to the stomach. These approaches can be administered before and during exercise and can also be combined – an approach that may be more beneficial (2).

The best way to induce meaningful reductions in physiological strain and improve subsequent prolonged exercise performance is to pre-cool the athlete using whole-body cold-water immersion. Explosive activities may be impaired if the temperature of the active muscles is reduced and so cold-water immersion prior to such exercise should be avoided. The benefits of pre-cooling are often lost or diminished during exercise (4–9) but cooling during exercise may extend the duration so that the participants experience a lower actual or perceived thermal strain. The most effective per-cooling interventions are less effective at lowering physiological strain than the most effective pre-cooling interventions because a balance needs to be struck between the magnitude of cooling offered and the practicality of the intervention. Commonly used per-cooling interventions include ice vests (4;11–13), neck cooling collars (14–17), and cold beverage/ice slurry ingestion (18;19). Cooling garments can improve exercise performance by reducing physiological and perceptual strain but care should be taken to ensure that the garment offers as much cooling as you think if physiological alterations are desired (as often these garments do not cool the entire surface that they cover). It is also important that their mass does not impede movement which would negate any benefit of the cooling. Drinking a cold or iced beverage prior to exercise can directly cool the tissues that the fluid comes into contact with (e.g. the mouth) but can also lower core body temperature and slow the rate at which it rises during exercise in the heat (7;18;23). Internal per-cooling does not consistently reduce core body temperature (18;19;103–105) because it can suppress the sudomotor response to heat, reducing sweat rate, sweat loss, and evaporative heat loss from the skin (23;30;100;103–106).

Less frequently used interventions include fan cooling and menthol application. Fan cooling can provide a convective cooling to the athlete and can be provided naturally (e.g. wind or airflow while cycling) or artificially (e.g. fan cooling substitutes while they are on the substitutes bench). Fan cooling can reduce physiological and perceptual strain (72;74;77;78), especially when accompanied with skin wetting to increase evaporative heat loss, and although it might impair short-duration cycling capacity (78) it consistently improves prolonged exercise performance and capacity. If reductions in physiological strain are not required, menthol cooling may be a practical option for your athletes. Menthol does not reduce physiological strain (83–86), but activates the same receptors (TRPM8) as cool air to give the sensation of cooling. It can be applied to the skin (usually as a gel or spray), rinsed in the mouth, or ingested (24;25;80–82), and its effectiveness appears to be dose-dependent (94;97). Menthol can improve exercise performance and capacity in the heat due to the sensation of cooling and subsequent improvements in thermal comfort.

When it comes to cooling your athlete, you need to decide what your objective is (is it to lower physiological strain? Is it to lower perceptual strain? Is it to do both?), thoroughly review the demands of the sport, and identify where cooling can be practically applied. In many cases, the best approach may not be feasible and so you need to pick the optimal approach/approaches for your specific athlete and situation.

7.6 Self-check quiz

At the start of this chapter you were told that by this point you should know the following:

- How and when athlete cooling strategies can be used
- The effect of different cooling approaches on exercise performance
- The effect of different cooling approaches on the physiological and perceptual response to exercise

This short self-check quiz will help you establish whether there are any areas of this chapter that need another look. Before looking at the answers, reread the following sections for assistance: Section 7.2 (questions 1–3) and Section 7.3 (questions 4–10).

7.6.1 Self-check quiz questions

1. When are pre- and per-cooling strategies used?
2. What is the main aim of pre-cooling an athlete?
3. What is mixed-method cooling?
4. What is the difference between internal cooling and external cooling?
5. What is the "after-drop" that is sometimes observed when using cold-water immersion to cool athletes?

6. What type of exercise is least likely to benefit from cold-water immersion pre-cooling?
7. Ice vests cover approximately 25% of the body surface area; however, due to their design, the surface area actually cooled is much lower. What percentage of the body surface area is actually cooled by most ice vests?
8. Name a practical way of providing convective cooling to an athlete
9. Is menthol an effective way to cool an athlete before or during exercise?
10. Why does internal cooling tend to use iced, rather than cold, drinks?

7.6.2 Self-check quiz answers

1. Pre-cooling strategies are used before exercise whereas per-cooling strategies are used during exercise.
2. To enable the athlete to start the exercise bout with a lower level of physiological and perceptual strain to enable them to either exercise for longer or to exercise harder.
3. Mixed-method cooling involves a combination of approaches, e.g. torso cooling, neck cooling, thigh cooling.
4. External cooling interventions attempt to reduce the actual and perceived levels of thermal strain experienced by directly cooling the skin, peripheral blood, and superficial tissues, whereas internal cooling directly cools the tissues from the oral cavity to the stomach.
5. A delayed reduction in core body temperature, which is caused by a restarting of peripheral blood flow once the athlete is removed from the cold water. When the athlete is immersed in the cold water, peripheral vasoconstriction occurs and this limits the movement of cool blood from the periphery to the core. Once the athlete is removed from the cold water, peripheral blood flow restarts and the cool peripheral blood circulates to the core cooling it down.
6. Sprint/explosive exercise using the large muscle groups.
7. 5–10%.
8. Providing airflow using a fan.
9. No. Menthol does not reduce physiological strain but activates the same receptors (transient receptor potential ion channel melastatin 8 (TRPM8 for short)) activated by air temperatures between 8°C and 28°C and so gives the sensation of cooling.
10. Drinking an ice slurry can approximately double the heat sink, compared to that created by drinking a cold beverage alone.

7.7 Practical toolkit

7.7.1 Cooling summary

Table 7.1a is a completed version of Table 7.1 and can be used as a quick reference guide to compare and contrast the commonly used cooling approaches.

TABLE 7.1A Table summarising the most commonly used cooling strategies (to be completed)

Cooling approach	Internal?	External?	Pre-cooling?	Per-cooling?	Pros	Cons
Whole-body cold-water immersion		✓	✓		Very large area cooled Effective at reducing physiological and perceptual strain	Impractical in many settings Causes disruption to pre-competition routines large area cooled
Lower body cold-water immersion		✓	✓		Very large area cooled Effective at reducing physiological and perceptual strain	Impractical in many settings Causes disruption to pre-competition routines large area cooled
Ice vest		✓	✓	✓	Covers a large surface area of the body Relatively inexpensive Can improve physiological and perceptual strain Practical for field use	Can be heavy and bulky Not all of the area covered is cooled Cooling power can be lost quickly
Cooling collar/hood		✓	✓	✓	Relatively inexpensive Improves perceived strain Practical for field use ✓	Only covers a small surface area of the body No effect on physiological strain May enable athletes to override "stop signals" Cooling power can be lost quickly
Fans and water spray		✓	✓	✓	Potentially a very large area cooled Relatively inexpensive Improves physiological and perceived strain Somewhat practical for field use	Requires electrical power
Ice/cold-water ingestion	✓		✓	✓	Practical for field use Can improve physiological and perceptual strain Inexpensive Tackles hypohydration	Potential for gastrointestinal discomfort Can delay sweat response use
Menthol	✓	✓	✓	✓	Can improve perceptual strain Practical for field use Inexpensive	Does not reduce physiological strain May enable athletes to override any "stop signals" perceptual strain

References

1 Périard JD, Racinais S, Timpka T, Dahlstrom O, Spreco A, Jacobsson J, et al. Strategies and factors associated with preparing for competing in the heat: a cohort study at the 2015 IAAF World Athletics Championships. *Br J Sports Med* 2017 Feb;51(4):264–70.

2 Bogerd N, Perret C, Bogerd CP, Rossi RM, Daanen HA. The effect of precooling intensity on cooling efficiency and exercise performance. *J Sports Sci* 2010 May;28(7):771–9.

3 Tyler CJ, Sunderland C, Cheung SS. The effect of cooling prior to and during exercise on exercise performance and capacity in the heat: a meta-analysis. *Br J Sports Med* 2015 Jan;49(1):7–13.

4 Arngrimsson SA, Petitt DS, Stueck MG, Jorgensen DK, Cureton KJ. Cooling vest worn during active warm-up improves 5-km run performance in the heat. *J Appl Physiol* 2004 May;96(5):1867–74.

5 Booth J, Marino FE, Ward JJ. Improved running performance in hot humid conditions following whole body precooling. *Med Sci Sports Exerc* 1997;29(7):943–9.

6 Duffield R, Green R, Castle P, Maxwell N. Precooling can prevent the reduction of self-paced exercise intensity in the heat. *Med Sci Sports Exerc* 2010 Mar;42(3):577–84.

7 Hasegawa H, Takatori T, Komura T, Yamasaki M. Combined effects of pre-cooling and water ingestion on thermoregulation and physical capacity during exercise in a hot environment. *J Sports Sci* 2006 Jan;24(1):3–9.

8 Kay D, Taaffe DR, Marino FE. Whole-body pre-cooling and heat storage during self-paced cycling performance in warm humid conditions. *J Sports Sci* 1999;17:937–44.

9 Quod MJ, Martin DT, Laursen PB, Gardner AS, Halson SL, Marino FE, et al. Practical precooling: effect on cycling time trial performance in warm conditions. *J Sports Sci* 2008 Dec;26(14):1477–87.

10 Ansley L, Marvin G, Sharma A, Kendall MJ, Jones DA, Bridge MW. The effects of head cooling on endurance and neuroendocrine responses to exercise in warm conditions. *Physiol Res* 2008;57(6):863–72.

11 Kenny GP, Schissler AR, Stapleton J, Piamonte M, Binder K, Lynn A, et al. Ice cooling vest on tolerance for exercise under uncompensable heat stress. *J Occup Environ Hyg* 2011 Aug;8(8):484–91.

12 Cuttell SA, Kiri V, Tyler C. A comparison of 2 practical cooling methods on cycling capacity in the heat. *J Athl Train* 2016 Aug 29;51(7):525–32.

13 Luomala MJ, Oksa J, Salmi JA, Linnamo V, Holmer I, Smolander J, et al. Adding a cooling vest during cycling improves performance in warm and humid conditions. *J Therm Biol* 2012;37:47–55.

14 Tyler CJ, Wild P, Sunderland C. Practical neck cooling and time-trial running performance in a hot environment. *Eur J Appl Physiol* 2010 Nov;110(5):1063–74.

15 Tyler CJ, Sunderland C. Neck cooling and running performance in the heat: single versus repeated application. *Med Sci Sports Exerc* 2011 Dec;43(12):2388–95.

16 Tyler CJ, Sunderland C. Cooling the neck region during exercise in the heat. *J Athl Train* 2011 Jan;46(1):61–8.

17 Lee JK, Koh AC, Koh SX, Liu GJ, Nio AQ, Fan PW. Neck cooling and cognitive performance following exercise-induced hyperthermia. *Eur J Appl Physiol* 2014 Feb;114(2):375–84.

18 Mundel T, King J, Collacott E, Jones DA. Drink temperature influences fluid intake and endurance capacity in men during exercise in a hot, dry environment. *Exp Physiol* 2006 Sep;91(5):925–33.

19 Schulze E, Daanen HA, Levels K, Casadio JR, Plews DJ, Kilding AE, et al. Effect of thermal state and thermal comfort on cycling performance in the heat. *Int J Sports Physiol Perform* 2015 Jul;10(5):655–63.

20 Stevens CJ, Taylor L, Dascombe BJ. Cooling during exercise: an overlooked strategy for enhancing endurance performance in the heat. *Sports Med* 2017 May;47(5):829–41.

21 Bongers CC, Hopman MT, Eijsvogels TM. Cooling interventions for athletes: an overview of effectiveness, physiological mechanisms, and practical considerations. *Temperature (Austin)* 2017;4(1):60–78.

22 Bongers CC, Thijssen DH, Veltmeijer MT, Hopman MT, Eijsvogels TM. Precooling and percooling (cooling during exercise) both improve performance in the heat: a meta-analytical review. *Br J Sports Med* 2015 Mar;49(6):377–84.

23 Lee JK, Shirreffs SM, Maughan RJ. Cold drink ingestion improves exercise endurance capacity in the heat. *Med Sci Sports Exerc* 2008 Sep;40(9):1637–44.

24 Riera F, Trong TT, Sinnapah S, Hue O. Physical and perceptual cooling with beverages to increase cycle performance in a tropical climate. *PLoS One* 2014;9(8):e103718.

25 Tran TT, Riera F, Rinaldi K, Briki W, Hue O. Ingestion of a cold temperature/menthol beverage increases outdoor exercise performance in a hot, humid environment. *PLoS One* 2015;10(4):e0123815.

26 Marsh D, Sleivert G. Effect of precooling on high intensity cycling performance. *Br J Sports Med* 1999 Dec;33(6):393–7.

27 Goosey-Tolfrey V, Swainson M, Boyd C, Atkinson G, Tolfrey K. The effectiveness of hand cooling at reducing exercise-induced hyperthermia and improving distance-race performance in wheelchair and able-bodied athletes. *J Appl Physiol (1985)* 2008 Jul;105(1):37–43.

28 Racinais S, Blonc S, Oksa J, Hue O. Does the diurnal increase in central temperature interact with pre-cooling or passive warm-up of the leg? *J Sci Med Sport* 2009 Jan;12(1):97–100.

29 Gonzalez-Alonso J, Teller C, Andersen SL, Jensen FB, Hyldig T, Nielsen B. Influence of body temperature on the development of fatigue during prolonged exercise in the heat. *J Appl Physiol* 1999 Mar;86(3):1032–9.

30 Siegel R, Mate J, Watson G, Nosaka K, Laursen PB. Pre-cooling with ice slurry ingestion leads to similar run times to exhaustion in the heat as cold water immersion. *J Sports Sci* 2012;30(2):155–65.

31 Sleivert GG, Cotter JD, Roberts WS, Febbraio MA. The influence of whole-body vs. torso pre-cooling on physiological strain and performance of high-intensity exercise in the heat. *Comp Biochem Physiol A Mol Integr Physiol* 2001 Apr;128(4):657–66.

32 Vaile J, Halson S, Gill N, Dawson B. Effect of cold water immersion on repeat cycling performance and thermoregulation in the heat. *J Sports Sci* 2008 Mar;26(5):431–40.

33 Tyler CJ, Reeve T, Cheung SS. Cold-induced vasodilation during single digit immersion in 0 degrees C and 8 degrees C water in men and women. *PLoS One* 2015;10(4):e0122592.

34 Sendowski I, Savourey G, Besnard Y, Bittel J. Cold induced vasodilatation and cardiovascular responses in humans during cold water immersion of various upper limb areas. *Eur J Appl Physiol Occup Physiol* 1997;75(6):471–7.

35 Bigland-Ritchie B, Thomas CK, Rice CL, Howarth JV, Woods JJ. Muscle temperature, contractile speed, and motoneuron firing rates during human voluntary contractions. *J Appl Physiol* 1992 Dec;73(6):2457–61.

36 Febbraio MA, Snow RJ, Stathis CG, Hargreaves M, Carey MF. Effect of heat stress on muscle energy metabolism during exercise. *J Appl Physiol* 1994 Dec;77(6):2827–31.

37 Yeargin SW, Casa DJ, McClung JM, Knight JC, Healey JC, Goss PJ, et al. Body cooling between two bouts of exercise in the heat enhances subsequent performance. *J Strength Cond Res* 2006 May;20(2):383–9.

38 Castle PC, Macdonald AL, Philp A, Webborn A, Watt PW, Maxwell NS. Precooling leg muscle improves intermittent sprint exercise performance in hot, humid conditions. *J Appl Physiol* 2006;100(4):1377–84.

39 Martin DT, Hahn A, Ryan-Tanner R, Yates K, Lee H, Smith JA. Ice jackets are cool. *Sport Science* 1998;2(4). Available from sportsci.org/jour/9804/dtm.html.

40 Eijsvogels TM, Bongers CC, Veltmeijer MT, Moen MH, Hopman M. Cooling during exercise in temperate conditions: impact on performance and thermoregulation. *Int J Sports Med* 2014 Sep;35(10):840–6.

41 Cureton KJ, Sparling PB, Evans BW, Johnson SM, Kong UD, Purvis JW. Effect of experimental alterations in excess weight on aerobic capacity and distance running performance. *Med Sci Sports* 1978;10(3):194–9.

42 Clarke ND, Maclaren DP, Reilly T, Drust B. Carbohydrate ingestion and pre-cooling improves exercise capacity following soccer-specific intermittent exercise performed in the heat. *Eur J Appl Physiol* 2011 Jul;111(7):1447–55.

43 Price MJ, Boyd C, Goosey-Tolfrey VL. The physiological effects of pre-event and midevent cooling during intermittent running in the heat in elite female soccer players. *Appl Physiol Nutr Metab* 2009 Oct;34(5):942–9.

44 Webster J, Holland EJ, Sleiverts G, Laing RM, Niven BE. A light-weight cooling vest enhances performance of athletes in the heat. *Ergonomics* 2005;48(7):821–37.

45 Ando S, Komiyama T, Sudo M, Kiyonaga A, Tanaka H, Higaki Y. The effects of temporal neck cooling on cognitive function during strenuous exercise in a hot environment: a pilot study. *BMC Res Notes* 2015 May 30;8:202.

46 Bulbulian R, Shapiro R, Murphy M, Levenhagen D. Effectiveness of a commercial head-neck cooling device. *J Strength Cond Res* 1999;13(3):198–205.

47 Gordon NF, Bogdanffy GM, Wilkinson J. Effect of a practical neck cooling device on core temperature during exercise. *Med Sci Sports Exerc* 1990 Apr;22(2):245–9.

48 Sunderland C, Stevens R, Everson B, Tyler CJ. Neck-cooling improves repeated sprint performance in the heat. *Front Physiol* 2015;6:314.

49 Nunneley SA, Troutman SJ, Jr., Webb P. Head cooling in work and heat stress. *Aerosp Med* 1971 Jan;42(1):64–8.

50 Zhu L, Diao C. Theoretical simulation of temperature distribution in the brain during mild hypothermia treatment for brain injury. *Med Biol Eng Comput* 2001 Nov;39(6):681–7.

51 Cabanac M. Selective brain cooling in humans: "fancy" or fact? *FASEB J* 1993 Sep;7(12):1143–6.

52 Nunneley SA, Nelson DA. Limitations on arteriovenous cooling of the blood supply to the human brain. *Eur J Appl Physiol Occup Physiol* 1994;69(6):474–9.

53 Brengelmann GL. Specialized brain cooling in humans? *FASEB J* 1993 Sep;7(12):1148–52.

54 Zhu L. Theoretical evaluation of contributions of heat conduction and countercurrent heat exchange in selective brain cooling in humans. *Ann Biomed Eng* 2000;28(3):269–77.

55 Sukstanskii AL, Yablonskiy DA. Theoretical limits on brain cooling by external head cooling devices. *Eur J Appl Physiol* 2007 Apr 12;101(1):41–9.

56 Nybo L, Moller K, Volianitis S, Nielsen B, Secher NH. Effects of hyperthermia on cerebral blood flow and metabolism during prolonged exercise in humans. *J Appl Physiol* 2002 Jul;93(1):58–64.

57 Shiraki K, Sagawa S, Tajima F, Yokota A, Hashimoto M, Brengelmann GL. Independence of brain and tympanic temperatures in an unanesthetized human. *J Appl Physiol* 1988 Jul;65(1):482–6.

58 Cotter JD, Taylor NA. The distribution of cutaneous sudomotor and alliesthesial thermosensitivity in mildly heat-stressed humans: an open-loop approach. *J Physiol* 2005 May 15;565(Pt 1):335–45.

59 Kissen AT, Hall JF, Jr., Klemm FK. Physiological responses to cooling the head and neck versus the trunk and leg areas in severe hyperthermic exposure. *Aerosp Med* 1971 Aug;42(8):882–8.

60 McCaffrey TV, Geis GS, Chung JM, Wurster RD. Effect of isolated head heating and cooling on sweating in man. *Aviat Space Environ Med* 1975 Nov;46(11):1353–7.

61 Shvartz E. Effect of a cooling hood on physiological responses to work in a hot environment. *J Appl Physiol* 1970 Jul;29(1):36–9.

62 Shvartz E. Effect of neck versus chest cooling on responses to work in heat. *J Appl Physiol* 1976 May;40(5):668–72.

63 Armada-da-Silva PA, Woods J, Jones DA. The effect of passive heating and face cooling on perceived exertion during exercise in the heat. *Eur J Appl Physiol* 2004 May;91(5–6):563–71.

64 Brown GA, Williams GM. The effect of head cooling on deep body temperature and thermal comfort in man. *Aviat Space Environ Med* 1982 Jun;53(6):583–6.

65 Hamada S, Torii M, Szygula Z, Adachi K. Effect of partial body cooling on thermophysiological responses during cycling work in a hot environment. *J Therm Biol* 2006;31:194–207.

66 Mundel T, Hooper P, Bunn S, Jones D. The effects of face-cooling on the perception of exertion and neuroendocrine response to hyperthermic exercise. *J Appl Physiol* 2005;565P:C31.

67 Palmer CD, Sleivert G, Cotter JD. The effects of head and neck cooling on thermoregulation, pace selection and performance. *Proc Aust Physiol Pharmacol Soc* 2001;32(2):122P.

68 Simmons SE, Mundel T, Jones DA. The effects of passive heating and head-cooling on perception of exercise in the heat. *Eur J Appl Physiol* 2008 Jan 3;271–80.

69 Tyler CJ, Wild P, Sunderland C. Practical neck cooling and time-trial running performance in a hot environment. *Eur J Appl Physiol* 2010 Aug 8;110(5):1063–74.

70 Tyler CJ, Sunderland C. Neck cooling and running performance in the heat: single versus repeated application. *Med Sci Sports Exerc* 2011 December; 43(12):2388–95.

71 Junge N, Jorgensen R, Flouris AD, Nybo L. Prolonged self-paced exercise in the heat – environmental factors affecting performance. *Temperature (Austin)* 2016;3(4):539–48.

72 Morrison SA, Cheung S, Cotter JD. Importance of airflow for physiologic and ergogenic effects of precooling. *J Athl Train* 2014 Sep;49(5):632–9.

73 Saunders AG, Dugas JP, Tucker R, Lambert MI, Noakes TD. The effects of different air velocities on heat storage and body temperature in humans cycling in a hot, humid environment. *Acta Physiol Scand* 2005 Mar;183(3):241–55.

74 Otani H, Kaya M, Tamaki A, Watson P, Maughan RJ. Air velocity influences thermoregulation and endurance exercise capacity in the heat. *Appl Physiol Nutr Metab* 2018 Feb;43(2):131–8.

75 Adams WC, Mack GW, Langhans GW, Nadel ER. Effects of varied air velocity on sweating and evaporative rates during exercise. *J Appl Physiol (1985)* 1992 Dec;73(6):2668–74.

76 Mora-Rodriguez R, del CJ, Aguado-Jimenez R, Estevez E. Separate and combined effects of airflow and rehydration during exercise in the heat. *Med Sci Sports Exerc* 2007 Oct;39(10):1720–6.

77 Schranner D, Scherer L, Lynch GP, Korder S, Brotherhood JR, Pluim BM, et al. In-play cooling interventions for simulated match-play tennis in hot/humid conditions. *Med Sci Sports Exerc* 2017 May;49(5):991–8.

78 Mitchell JB, McFarlin BK, Dugas JP. The effect of pre-exercise cooling on high intensity running performance in the heat. *Int J Sports Med* 2003 Feb;24(2):118–24.

79 Lynch GP, Periard JD, Pluim BM, Brotherhood JR, Jay O. Optimal cooling strategies for players in Australian Tennis Open conditions. *J Sci Med Sport* 2018 Mar;21(3):232–7.

80 Mundel T, Jones DA. The effects of swilling an L(-)-menthol solution during exercise in the heat. *Eur J Appl Physiol* 2010 May;109(1):59–65.

81 Stevens CJ, Thoseby B, Sculley DV, Callister R, Taylor L, Dascombe BJ. Running performance and thermal sensation in the heat are improved with menthol mouth rinse but not ice slurry ingestion. *Scand J Med Sci Sports* 2016 Oct;26(10):1209–16.

82 Stevens CJ, Bennett KJ, Sculley DV, Callister R, Taylor L, Dascombe BJ. A comparison of mixed-method cooling interventions on preloaded running performance in the heat. *J Strength Cond Res* 2017 Mar;31(3):620–9.

83 Barwood MJ, Corbett J, White D, James J. Early change in thermal perception is not a driver of anticipatory exercise pacing in the heat. *Br J Sports Med* 2012 Oct;46(13):936–42.

84 Barwood MJ, Corbett J, White DK. Spraying with 0.20% L-menthol does not enhance 5 km running performance in the heat in untrained runners. *J Sports Med Phys Fitness* 2014 Oct;54(5):595–604.

85 Barwood MJ, Corbett J, Thomas K, Twentyman P. Relieving thermal discomfort: effects of sprayed L-menthol on perception, performance, and time trial cycling in the heat. *Scand J Med Sci Sports* 2015 Jun;25(Suppl 1):211–8.

86 Schlader ZJ, Simmons SE, Stannard SR, Mundel T. The independent roles of temperature and thermal perception in the control of human thermoregulatory behavior. *Physiol Behav* 2011 May 3;103(2):217–24.

87 Montell C, Caterina MJ. Thermoregulation: channels that are cool to the core. *Curr Biol* 2007 Oct 23;17(20):R885–R887.

88 Tajino K, Hosokawa H, Maegawa S, Matsumura K, Dhaka A, Kobayashi S. Cooling-sensitive TRPM8 is thermostat of skin temperature against cooling. *PLoS One* 2011 Mar 2;6(3):e17504.

89 Green BG. The sensory effects of L-menthol on human skin. *Somatosens Mot Res* 1992;9(3):235–44.

90 Hatem S, Attal N, Willer JC, Bouhassira D. Psychophysical study of the effects of topical application of menthol in healthy volunteers. *Pain* 2006 May;122(1–2):190–6.

91 Gillis DJ, House JR, Tipton MJ. The influence of menthol on thermoregulation and perception during exercise in warm, humid conditions. *Eur J Appl Physiol* 2010 Oct;110(3):609–18.

92 Schlader ZJ, Simmons SE, Stannard SR, Mundel T. The independent roles of temperature and thermal perception in the control of human thermoregulatory behavior. *Physiol Behav* 2011 May; 103(2):217–24.

93 Gillis DJ, Barwood MJ, Newton PS, House JR, Tipton MJ. The influence of a menthol and ethanol soaked garment on human temperature regulation and perception during exercise and rest in warm, humid conditions. *J Therm Biol* 2016 May;58:99–105.

94 Kounalakis SN, Botonis PG, Koskolou MD, Geladas ND. The effect of menthol application to the skin on sweating rate response during exercise in swimmers and controls. *Eur J Appl Physiol* 2010 May;109(2):183–9.

95 Johnson CD, Melanaphy D, Purse A, Stokesberry SA, Dickson P, Zholos AV. Transient receptor potential melastatin 8 channel involvement in the regulation of vascular tone. *Am J Physiol Heart Circ Physiol* 2009 Jun;296(6):H1868–H1877.

96 Yosipovitch G, Szolar C, Hui XY, Maibach H. Effect of topically applied menthol on thermal, pain and itch sensations and biophysical properties of the skin. *Arch Dermatol Res* 1996 May;288(5–6):245–8.

97 Tajino K, Matsumura K, Kosada K, Shibakusa T, Inoue K, Fushiki T, et al. Application of menthol to the skin of whole trunk in mice induces autonomic and behavioral heat-gain responses. *Am J Physiol Regul Integr Comp Physiol* 2007 Nov;293(5):R2128–R2135.

98 Ihsan M, Landers G, Brearley M, Peeling P. Beneficial effects of ice ingestion as a precooling strategy on 40-km cycling time-trial performance. *Int J Sports Physiol Perform* 2010 Jun;5(2):140–51.

99 Stanley J, Leveritt M, Peake JM. Thermoregulatory responses to ice-slush beverage ingestion and exercise in the heat. *Eur J Appl Physiol* 2010 Dec;110(6):1163–73.

100 Zimmermann M, Landers G, Wallman KE, Saldaris J. The effects of crushed ice ingestion prior to steady state exercise in the heat. *Int J Sport Nutr Exerc Metab* 2017 Jun;27(3):220–7.

101 Snipe RMJ, Costa RJS. Does the temperature of water ingested during exertional-heat stress influence gastrointestinal injury, symptoms, and systemic inflammatory profile? *J Sci Med Sport* 2018 Jan 8;21(1):771–6.

102 Burdon C, O'Connor H, Gifford J, Shirreffs S, Chapman P, Johnson N. Effect of drink temperature on core temperature and endurance cycling performance in warm, humid conditions. *J Sports Sci* 2010 Sep;28(11):1147–56.

103 Burdon CA, Hoon MW, Johnson NA, Chapman PG, O'Connor HT. The effect of ice slushy ingestion and mouthwash on thermoregulation and endurance performance in the heat. *Int J Sport Nutr Exerc Metab* 2013 Oct;23(5):458–69.

104 Lee JK, Maughan RJ, Shirreffs SM. The influence of serial feeding of drinks at different temperatures on thermoregulatory responses during cycling. *J Sports Sci* 2008 Apr;26(6):583–90.

105 Morris NB, Coombs G, Jay O. Ice slurry ingestion leads to a lower net heat loss during exercise in the heat. *Med Sci Sports Exerc* 2016 Jan;48(1):114–22.

106 Jay O, Morris NB. Does cold water or ice slurry ingestion during exercise elicit a net body cooling effect in the heat? *Sports Med* 2018 Jan 24;48(Suppl 1):17–29.

107 Morris NB, Bain AR, Cramer MN, Jay O. Evidence that transient changes in sudomotor output with cold and warm fluid ingestion are independently modulated by abdominal, but not oral thermoreceptors. *J Appl Physiol (1985)* 2014 Apr 15;116(8):1088–95.

108 Siegel R, Laursen PB. Keeping your cool: possible mechanisms for enhanced exercise performance in the heat with internal cooling methods. *Sports Med* 2012 Feb 1;42(2):89–98.

109 Cotter JD, Sleivert GG, Roberts WS, Febbraio MA. Effect of pre-cooling, with and without thigh cooling, on strain and endurance exercise performance in the heat. *Comp Biochem Physiol A Mol Integr Physiol* 2001 Apr;128(4):667–77.

110 Minett GM, Duffield R, Kellett A, Portus M. Mixed-method pre-cooling reduces physiological demand without improving performance of medium-fast bowling in the heat. *J Sports Sci* 2012 May;30(9):907–15.

111 Minett GM, Duffield R, Marino FE, Portus M. Duration-dependant response of mixed-method pre-cooling for intermittent-sprint exercise in the heat. *Eur J Appl Physiol* 2012 Feb 17.

112 Minett GM, Duffield R, Marino FE, Portus M. Volume-dependent response of precooling for intermittent-sprint exercise in the heat. *Med Sci Sports Exerc* 2011 Sep;43(9):1760–9.

113 Gaoua N, Racinais S, Grantham J, El MF. Alterations in cognitive performance during passive hyperthermia are task dependent. *Int J Hyperthermia* 2011;27(1):1–9.

114 Bandelow S, Maughan RJ, Shirreffs SM, Ozgunen K, Kurdak S, Ersoz G, et al. The effects of exercise, heat, cooling and rehydration strategies on cognitive function in football players. *Scand J Med Sci Sports* 2010;20(3):148–60.

115 Racinais S, Gaoua N, Grantham J. Hyperthermia impairs short-term memory and peripheral motor drive transmission. *J Physiol* 2008 Oct 1;586(Pt 19):4751–62.

116 Simmons SE, Saxby BK, McGlone FP, Jones DA. The effect of passive heating and head cooling on perception, cardiovascular function and cognitive performance in the heat. *Eur J Appl Physiol* 2008 Sep;104(2):271–80.

117 Nunneley SA, Reader DC, Maldonado RJ. Head-temperature effects on physiology, comfort, and performance during hyperthermia. *Aviat Space Environ Med* 1982 Jul;53(7):623–8.

8

(DE)HYDRATION

What should you know by the end of the chapter?

The topic of dehydration is one frequently discussed in the scientific literature and in the popular media. This chapter will look at the effects that reductions in body water content have on the body and exercise performance. By the end of this chapter you should be able to answer questions related to the following:

- Is maintaining hydration status important for an athlete?
- Does hydration status influence exercise performance?
- How can you assess hydration status and what is the best approach?
- What are the physiological responses to hypohydration?
- Are there any risks to over-hydrating?

Key terms for this chapter

Aldosterone
A steroid hormone that regulates the reabsorption of sodium. If aldosterone is lacking, there will be a high concentration of sodium in the urine.

Arginine vasopressin
A peptide hormone whose primary function is to regulate extracellular fluid volume. Arginine vasopressin (often abbreviated to AVP) acts on renal collecting ducts to increase water permeability and decrease urine formation. Due to the decrease in diuresis, it is also referred to as antidiuretic hormone (ADH).

Dehydration
The process of losing water – either from a hyperhydrated state to a euhydrated one or from a euhydrated state to a hypohydrated one.

Hyperhydration
A fluid-induced state in which body mass is at least 0.22% greater than normal in temperate conditions and at least

0.48% greater than normal in hot conditions (or during exercise).

Hypertonic fluid — A fluid with a higher osmolality than a comparative solution (usually plasma).

Hypohydration — A fluid-induced state in which body mass is at least 0.22% lower than normal in temperate conditions and at least 0.48% lower than normal in hot conditions (or during exercise) (plasma osmolality ≥290 mOsmol (1)). Hypohydration runs on a continuum with 2–5% reductions being referred to as mild to moderate and >5% being referred to as severe in athletic populations (2).

Hyponatremia — A blood, serum, or plasma sodium concentration below 135 mmol·L^{-1} often caused by the overconsumption of water.

Hypotonic fluid — A fluid with a lower osmolality than a comparative solution (usually plasma).

Euhydration — A state of fluid balance (plasma osmolality of 280–290 mOsmol (1)).

Isotonic fluid — A fluid with an identical osmolality to a comparative solution (usually plasma).

Osmolality — The number of osmoles per unit of solution – a larger value represents a greater concentration. Plasma osmolality is considered the "gold standard" approach for hydration assessment but urine osmolality is also used.

Refractometer — A device for the measurement of an index of light refraction – can be used to measure urine specific gravity.

Rehydration — The process of gaining water from a hypohydrated state towards a euhydrated one.

Problem 8.1: Assessment of hydration status in the field

You are a sport scientist working for a local athletics club and wish to begin a programme of hydration monitoring with your athletes. You have a budget of £200 for this and see each athlete twice a week. Which method, or methods, would you use? Why?

Problem 8.2: Optimising hydration for the team sport athlete

You are a sports scientist working for a semi-professional football club. You have a busy pre-season period coming up and the weather is going to be warm (28–35°C). What hydration strategies should you adopt?

8.1 Basics of fluid balance regulation

8.1.1 Total body water

Typical total body water makes up ~60% of nude body mass, but the percentage can range from 45% to 75% due to differences in body composition. Fat-free mass is predominately water (70–80%) whereas adipose tissue is ~10% water, and so total body water will make up a higher percentage of total body mass in leaner individuals. Total body water is split between intra- and extracellular compartments of the body with most of it being located in the intracellular spaces (~65%). Of the extracellular fluid, ~20% is plasma volume and ~80% is interstitial fluid.

Quick question: Maintaining water balance (euhydration) requires an athlete to have equal fluid losses and gains. How many ways can you think of that an athlete can gain or lose fluid?

Fluid can be gained from eating (diet-dependent), drinking (diet-dependent), and metabolism (~250–350 ml·d^{-1}), and lost by respiration (~250–350 ml·d^{-1}), sweating (~450–3,600 ml·d^{-1} depending on the environmental conditions and activity intensity), defaecating (~100–200 ml·d^{-1}), and urinating (~500–1,000 ml·d^{-1}). During exercise in the heat, urinary output is decreased but hypohydration still frequently occurs due to a failure to replace the fluid lost as sweat. The failure to replace the lost fluid might be due to deliberate fluid restriction (e.g. to avoid slowing down during a marathon race to pick up a water bottle from a drinks station or to "make weight" for a weight-classification sport) or unintentional due to the difficulty in taking fluids in during the activity (e.g. in a sport without many natural breaks in play).

Hydration status fluctuates throughout the day in a sinusoidal manner – moving between states of hyper- or hypo-hydration. Hyperhydration describes a fluid-induced state in which body mass is at least 0.22% greater than normal in temperate conditions and at least 0.48% greater than normal in hot conditions (or during exercise) while hypohydration describes body mass lower than normal by 0.22% and 0.48% in temperate and hot conditions (or during exercise), respectively (3).

8.1.2 Dehydration and rehydration

Quick question: "Dehydration" is word used frequently in the media – what does the word mean to you?

Dehydration is the process of losing water – either from a hyperhydrated state to a euhydrated one or from a euhydrated state to a hypohydrated one. "Dehydration" is usually used to describe whole-body fluid loss but it can be broken down into the same two subcategories that total body water can be broken down into – intra- and extracellular dehydration. Intracellular dehydration describes a loss of fluid from within the cell. Intracellular dehydration dries out the cell and increases blood sodium concentrations or osmolality. Extracellular dehydration describes the osmotic movement of fluid from outside the cell into the intracellular spaces which causes a reduction in plasma volume (hypovolaemia) due to a loss in sodium from the extracellular space. Rehydration is simply the opposite of dehydration – it is (intra- and extracellular) the process of gaining water from a hypohydrated state towards a euhydrated one.

8.1.3 Thirst

Thirst is a sensation defined as a desire to drink due to a deficit of water (3), and is stimulated by changes in plasma osmolality and changes in pressure.

1. Changes in plasma osmolality: Increased effective osmolality of the extracellular fluid causes intracellular dehydration which is detected by osmoreceptors located in the anterior hypothalamus.
2. Changes in pressure. Intravascular hypovolaemia caused by losses in extracellular fluid is detected by baroreceptors located in the cardiac atria (4).

Increases in plasma osmolality is the primary driver because an increase of only 1–4% (the threshold is highly variable between individuals) is required to initiate the sensation of thirst whereas far greater extracellular fluid reductions (10–15%) are required to cause thirst through the second pathway (4–6). Thirst is stimulated when plasma osmolality rises and arginine vasopressin is released (7) but is suppressed prior to changes in plasma osmolality when fluid is consumed (8). Suppression in the thirst sensation does not align with plasma osmolality but it does with reductions in plasma arginine vasopressin concentrations (8) in what appears to be a sophisticated mechanism to prevent over-hydrating by taking into consideration the time required for the gastrointestinal absorption of water. In contrast, osmoreceptors located in the gut (9) and oropharyngeal region can trigger sensations of thirst satiety before a sufficient volume of fluid has been consumed (10;11) which can lead to involuntary hypohydration, (especially when fluid is consumed without food) and so fluid should not be consumed too rapidly.

Thirst is subjective and difficult to quantify but can be assessed using either a visual analogue scale or a categorical scale. Visual analogue scales used to assess thirst are accompanied by a question such as "How thirsty do you feel now?" and are anchored by opposing statements such as "not thirsty" or "not at all thirsty" and "very thirsty" or "extremely thirsty". The person completing the assessment makes a mark on the line of known length (e.g. 10 cm) and this is measured and converted into a numerical value (12) e.g. a mark made at 6.2 cm is converted into a score of 6.2 out of 10.

The original thirst sensation scale was a comprehensive 37 item survey assessing a range of feelings, symptoms, and sensations related to thirst. Due to the time required to complete the thirst sensation scale, simplified versions have been produced. Some are non-numerical (e.g. Phillips et al. (13), who ask patients to rate thirst on a four-point scale: none, mild, moderate, and severe) but others have a number attached – probably the most commonly used categorical scale is the nine-point scale devised by Engell et al. (14) which ranges from 1 ("not thirsty") to 9 ("very thirsty").

8.2 Measurement of hydration status

This section will help you with Problem 8.1: Assessment of hydration status in the field: "You are a sport scientist working for a local athletics club and wish to

TABLE 8.1 Summary of ways to measure hydration status

	Units	Invasive?	Normal range	Hypohydrated if:	Pros	Cons
Urine specific gravity		Somewhat[a]	1.005–1.030	≥1.020		
Plasma osmolality	mOsmol	Yes	280–290	≥290		
Urine osmolality	mOsmol	Somewhat[a]	300–900	≥700		
Body mass change	kg	No	<0.2% BM	>0.2% BM		
Urine colour	1–8	Somewhat[a]	<4	>4		

a   Some athletes may be self-conscious about providing a urine sample.

begin a programme of hydration monitoring with your athletes – you have a budget of £200 for this. You see each athlete twice a week. Which method, or methods, would you use? Why?"

Fluid intake and losses are episodic and so the total body water volume fluctuates throughout the day. Fluctuations in total body water are usually small, but they can be large during periods of heat exposure and/or exercise. There are a number of ways to assess hydration status, the most commonly adopted hydration assessment strategies and thresholds are summarised in Table 8.1.

Quick question: You will see that the pros and cons columns in Table 8.1 are currently empty. You will be able to complete the table by the end of this section (Table 8.1a) but before you do, can you think of any pros and/or cons now?

Each method of assessing hydration status has strengths and weaknesses but, regardless of the method used, pre-measurement standardisation is crucial in order to be able to make meaningful inferences from your data. Such standardisation procedures should include:

- Completing the measurement at the same time of day on each occasion
- Using the same equipment for each assessment
- Standardising diet/exercise/sleep prior to assessment
- Ensuring that the same investigator completes the analysis

8.2.1 Osmolality of plasma and urine

Osmolality measures the number of osmoles of a solute per unit of solvent (e.g. $osmol \cdot kg^{-1}$) whereas osmolarity is the number of osmoles per unit of solution (e.g. $osmol \cdot l^{-1}$). Osmolality and osmolarity both measure concentrations and so a larger value represents a greater concentration. When it comes to hydration assessment, plasma osmolality is considered the "gold standard" approach but

TABLE 8.1A Quick reference table – reference values, and pros and cons of the most commonly used hydration assessment techniques

	Units	Invasive?	Normal range	Hypohydrated if:	Pros	Cons
Urine specific gravity		Somewhat[a]	1.005–1.030	≥1.020	Quick, simple, and easy to use in the field and in the lab Relatively inexpensive equipment needed	Unable to detect acute changes
Plasma osmolality	mOsmol	Yes	275–290	≥290	Accurate and reliable	Complex, expensive, and invasive
Urine osmolality	mOsmol	Somewhat[a]	300–900	≥700	More physiologically accurate than other urinary measures Quick, simple, and easy to use in the field and in the lab Inexpensive equipment needed	Low agreement with plasma values Requires specialist equipment
Body mass change	kg	No	<0.2% BM	>0.2% BM		Variable Confounded by changes in body composition
Urine colour	1–8	Somewhat[a]	<4	>4	Quick, simple, and easy to use in the field and in the laboratory Very inexpensive equipment needed	Subjective measurement Urine colour can be affected by other factors e.g. diet

a   Some athletes may be self-conscious about providing a urine sample.

urine osmolality is also used. Osmolality is measured using an osmometer, and the freezing point depression of water technique.

Plasma osmolality is the best way to assess changes in hydration status caused by sweat loss (15) because sweat contains a number of electrolytes (primarily sodium) that are hypotonic relative to plasma meaning that sweat-mediated hypohydration increases plasma osmolality. When using plasma osmolality, euhydration is defined as an osmolality of 280–290 mOsmol (1). Assessing plasma osmolality is invasive as it requires the drawing of blood and so midstream urinary assessment is sometimes used with a euhydration cut-off of <700 mOsmol. Urine osmolality is much more variable than plasma osmolality but it is physiologically more accurate than other urinary measures (see below) because it is unaffected by other solutes e.g. glucose. While plasma osmolality is the best way of assessing sweat-mediated hypohydration, there are no valid measurements of hypohydration caused by altitude, cold, diuretics, vomiting, or secretory diarrhoea that induce isotonic, rather than hypertonic, hypovolaemia (16).

8.2.2 Urine specific gravity

Urine specific gravity (USG) is a measure of the density of urine compared to the density of water (specific gravity of water = 1.000) and normally ranges between 1.003 and 1.035 with euhydration often being defined as a USG value of between 1.010 and 1.020 (17). In order to measure USG, an athlete provides a midstream urine sample, which is then analysed using a handheld refractometer. The refractometer measures the amount of substance dissolved in the urine using the principle of light refraction through liquids i.e. as light passes from air into a liquid it slows down. The more dissolved solids present in the urine, the slower light will travel through it. USG has a moderate relationship with plasma osmolality ($r = 0.46$) (18), and urine osmolality ($r = 0.64$) (19); however, USG often underestimates hydration status. In a study by Hew-Butler et al. (19), 27% of participants were classified as hypohydrated using the USG cut-off of ≥1.020 but 55% were classified as hypohydrated when classified using urine osmolality.

8.2.3 Urine colour

Armstrong et al. (20) sought a cheap and practical way to assess hydration status, and so devised a colour scale to assess urine colour as a marker of hydration status. The scale ranges from 1 ("very pale yellow", the lightest colour indicating very well hydrated) to 8 ("brownish green", the darkest colour indicating extremely dehydrated). Despite the indirect, and subjective ("is that a 4 or a 5?"), nature of using urine colour as a marker of hydration status, an athlete with a urine colour of 5 is nearly 6 times more likely to be hypohydrated than an individual with urine at a 4 or less on the chart (21). A urine colour of greater than 5 identifies hypohydration (induced by exercise in the heat) with a diagnostic accuracy of 87% (21) and so in many applied cases this form assessment is acceptable.

Armstrong et al. (20) proposed that athletes should aim to maintain urine that is "very pale yellow", "pale yellow", or "straw-coloured", which corresponds to 1, 2, and 3 on their urine colour chart, respectively. While maintaining such a colour may be an indicator of euhydration, copious dilute urinary excretion may be reflective of arginine vasopressin suppression (as a result of fluid intake in excess of osmoregulatory need (4)), and so drinking to keep urine clear may lead to hyperhydration (22). Urine colour assessed using the scale devised by Armstrong et al. (20) is well correlated with urine osmolality ($r = 0.82$) and USG ($r = 0.80$); however, outliers in the data highlight that colour should not be used when precise and accurate data are required. It is also worth noting that the colour of your urine colour can be influenced by non-hydration-related factors, such as diet and medication, and so standardisation is key to facilitate meaningful comparisons.

8.2.4 Body mass change

A first morning, post-urination, body mass will usually vary by less than 1% for a well-hydrated athlete in energy balance (23;24), and so measuring body mass is a cheap, easy way to estimate hydration status on a day-to-day basis. Change in body mass gives an estimation of fluid balance changes (e.g. a 2% loss of body mass is a good indicator of a 3% drop in total body water (24)) but it does not give any indication of where the fluid has been lost from. Measurements should be made on at least three consecutive days to establish a baseline value from which to evaluate deviations (23). For female athletes, the phase of the menstrual cycle at which measurements are taken should be considered as body mass can fluctuate throughout the cycle (25), and so practitioners should take care to ensure that like-for-like comparisons are being made.

Pre- and post-exercise body mass measurements are routinely used to estimate sweat loss and sweat rates within sessions based on the assumption that a decrease in body mass of 1 g is equal to 1 ml of sweat lost. Below you will see a worked example based on the following pre- and post-session body mass measurements (Toolbox 8.2 contains the equations for these estimations):

Pre-session body mass	84.1 kg
Post-session body mass	82.8 kg
Change in body mass (post-session body mass − pre-session body mass)	−1.3 kg
Estimated sweat loss (−1 g = −1 ml)	−1,300 ml
Session duration	120 min
Estimated sweat rate (estimated sweat loss/session duration)	650 ml·h^{-1}

Nude body mass should be used where possible, because otherwise sweat in the clothing will result in an overestimation of post-session body mass and an underestimation of sweat loss. Overestimations of 5–15% (26) in sweat loss can occur by ignoring respiratory water loss and carbon exchange (27); however, their assessment is complex and so as long as all other considerations are standardised, pre- and post-session mass changes will give a good estimation of sweat loss.

8.2.5 Clinical variables

Blood and urine markers are often impractical for large-scale assessment, and some practitioners have claimed that hydration status can be estimated using clinical examination of variables such as skin turgor (is the skin taut?), oral mucous membranes, the eye socket appearance (are the eyes sunken?), spit ability, and thirst sensation. While attractive from a time perspective, data show that these clinical assessment markers are unable to accurately detect body mass losses of >3% (28) and so they should not be used.

8.3 Physiological effects of hypohydration

Core body temperature is elevated when an athlete is hypohydrated due to a progressive decrease in whole-body sweating (29) and an increase in the threshold for sweat onset (i.e. you start sweating at a higher core body temperature than normal). The typical increase in core body temperature is approximately 0.1–0.2°C for every 1% hypohydration (30). Strenuous or prolonged exercise in the heat increases heart rate and total peripheral resistance while decreasing blood volume, mean arterial pressure, stroke volume, cardiac output, active and non-active limb blood flow, skin blood flow, and cerebral blood flow (31) (see Chapter 2 for more detail). Becoming hypohydrated places a further strain on the cardiovascular system of the exercising athlete because plasma is a major source of the fluid lost as sweat during exercise in the heat (32), and so as we sweat, plasma volume decreases. This reduction in plasma volume decreases total blood volume and stroke volume, and so heart rate must increase to maintain cardiac output – a response termed cardiovascular drift. The reduction in stroke volume observed when hypohydrated is likely to be due to reduction in cardiac filling time that occurs due to the increased heart rate and a decreased venous return. The increased heart rate decreases the time between beats, and as such, the window of opportunity for refilling whereas the lower venous return reduces the left ventricular end-diastolic volume (33). The cardiovascular strain observed when hyperthermic and hypohydrated can be reversed with fluid intake (34;35)

Two hormones are primarily involved in the regulation of body water balance – aldosterone and arginine vasopressin. Unless body water is excessive due to heavy sweating, these two hormones can usually maintain fluid and electrolyte balance within ~1% of normal levels. If osmoreceptors in the anterior hypothalamus detect an increase in plasma osmolality of ~2%, a compensatory release in arginine vasopressin from the posterior pituitary (in addition to an increase in thirst and renal water conservation) is initiated (9). Arginine vasopressin interacts with arginine vasopressin V_2 receptors in the kidney to increase the amount of water reabsorbed by the nephrons and reduce the volume of urine output. When hypohydration occurs, renal water compensation is unable to restore fluid balance and fluid intake must occur to restore fluid balance. Arginine vasopressin concentrations can also change in response to alterations in blood volume caused by changes in posture and skin blood flow (36) but very large blood volume reductions (in excess of 10% (~ 0.5 L)) are required. The release of arginine vasopressin often occurs simultaneously with the release of aldosterone. Hypohydration increases plasma aldosterone concentrations (37) by initiating the secretion of aldosterone from the adrenal glands. The increase in aldosterone increases sodium reabsorption in the kidney, which increases the osmolality of the blood and causes water to move from the extracellular to the intracellular spaces by osmosis and down a concentration gradient.

8.4 Effects of hypohydration on exercise performance in the heat

As discussed in Chapter 4, exercise performance is impaired in the heat due to a greater physiological and perceptual strain. The physiological and perceptual strain is exacerbated by hypohydration (Table 8.2) and so it seems prudent to suggest that hypohydration impairs performance but this is an area of debate. As ambient temperatures increase, the negative effect of hypohydration on exercise performance appears to become more pronounced and there is a noticeable impairment once skin temperature reaches 27.3°C (38). Sawka et al. (39) reported that hypohydration did not impair exercise in cool (2°C and 10°C; impairment observed in 0/2 studies) conditions, sometimes impaired exercise in temperate (20–24°C; 4/7 studies) conditions, and usually impaired exercise when it was hot (>25°C; 8/9 studies).

TABLE 8.2 The effect of hypohydration on physiological strain

Variable	Effect of hypohydration	Reason
Body temperature	↑	↑ sweat onset = ↓ sweat loss
		↓ skin blood flow = ↓ heat loss
Cardiac output	↓	↓ central blood volume = ↓ stroke volume
Cerebral blood flow	↓	↑ body temperature = ↑ hyperventilation = ↓ partial pressure of carbon dioxide in arterial blood
Heart rate	↑	↓ central blood volume = ↓ stroke volume
Limb blood flow	↓	↓ stroke volume = ↓ cardiac output
Mean arterial pressure	↓	↓ central blood volume
Skin blood flow	↓	↓ central blood volume and mean arterial pressure
Sweat loss	↓	↑ sweat onset
Sweat onset	↑	Conserve fluid
Stroke volume	↓	↑ heart rate = ↓ cardiac filling time
		↓ blood volume = ↓ mean arterial pressure = ↓ venous return
Urinary output	↓	↑ arginine vasopressin and aldosterone = ↑ water retention

Much of the data suggesting that exercise performance is impaired by hypohy-dration come from well-controlled laboratory studies and these led to the Ameri-can College of Sports Medicine recommending that fluid loss should be restricted to less than 2% to prevent impairing exercise performance. It has been proposed that strength and power tasks are unaffected by hypohydration but endurance ex-ercise is impaired when water deficient is greater than 3% (40) but meta-analysis data suggest that muscle endurance, strength, and anaerobic power are all impaired by hypohydration (41). Some of the discrepancy may be due to the grouping of similar, but different, research studies and the effects of hypohydration may depend on the nature of the protocol used. Hypohydration of ≤4% can have no effect on time-trial performance (and when comparing hypohydration of <2% with hypo-hydration of >2% there is no difference) but hypohydration levels as low as 1.75% can impair time-to-exhaustion, fixed-intensity exercise capacity tests (42).

Those that refute the suggestion that hypohydration impairs exercise perfor-mance often cite real-world data that show that successful runners tend to be very hypohydrated at the end of a race (43). There is an inverse relationship between body mass loss and performance time in a number of events, e.g. marathon running (44), ironman triathlon (45), and 24 h ultramarathon running (46) meaning that faster runners do finish the race more hypohydrated than their slower rivals (43) but it does not say that they run faster because they are hypohydrated (remember, correlation does not always equal causation!). These data are not new observations, with Pugh et al. (47) reporting that the first four finishers of a marathon held in 1966 lost an average of 5.8% of their body mass with the winner losing 6.9%. These body mass losses are far greater than the 2% suggested as impactful of performance, but nothing compared to the body mass that Haile Gebrselassie lost while winning the 2009 Dubai Marathon – he reportedly lost a whopping 9.8% (48)!

These data and the relationship between hydration status and exercise perfor-mance do not mean that hypohydration is good for exercise performance although it has been suggested that hypohydration-induced reductions in body mass might be beneficial for weight-dependent sports and activities such as vertical jumping (41). What these data suggest is that in order to be successful in those activities, ath-letes must be able to tolerate such a level of acute hypohydration – what is optimal is unknown. These data are often reported in well-trained individuals, and this may have a bearing on the conclusions drawn. For example, exercise performance impairments are ~1.75-fold greater in untrained individuals (41) and familiarising participants to a hypohydrated state appears to abolish performance impairments (49). Another factor that may impact upon the effect that hypohydration has on subsequent performance is the method of inducing the hypohydrated state with active dehydration protocols, increasing the impairments approximately two-fold compared to passive approaches (41). This has obvious implications for athletes.

Whether hypohydration impairs exercise performance or not is likely to be individual- and sport-specific and a more pertinent question might be "what is the optimal hydration status for a given athlete/event?" For example, as men-tioned, Haile Gebrselassie reportedly lost nearly 10% of his body mass while running the 2009 Dubai Marathon (48). At a pace of 4:47 min mile^{-1}, he was unlikely to be able to tolerate too much fluid without experiencing gastric discomfort and probably unwilling to stop/slow down to consume more fluid at each water station, as this would jeopardise his chances of winning.

Whether hypohydration has an effect on exercise performance appears to depend on a number of factors. These include:

- The ambient conditions – hotter conditions may exacerbate any negative effect of hypohydration
- The relevance of body mass to sporting success – is being lighter an advantage?
- Sport-specific demands – it is more difficult to take on fluid while running than stationary
- The training status of the individual – well-trained athletes may tolerate hypohydration better
- The level of familiarity the athlete has with being hypohydrated
- Whether the hypohydration is acute or chronic – most studies investigate acute hypohydration and so data on the long-term effects are limited

Despite years' worth of research, the question of whether hypohydration really impairs exercise performance is still heavily debated. As mentioned previously, for an athlete the answer is likely to be situation- and individual-specific, but research studies cannot cover all possible situational options and so often provide a conclusion based on the specific nature of the study designed. Hypohydration studies are tricky to design because often participants are not blinded to the intervention – for example, they know whether they are drinking or not – and this might have a large effect on the data recorded (especially performance data).

Quick question: How do you think you can blind study participants from knowing whether or not they are euhydrated?

Researchers have started to use two intravenous infusion (just like when you are hooked up to a drip at the hospital) and gastric tubes (a tube that is inserted down the throat into the stomach) to try to remove any potential placebo/nocebo effect of the participants knowing their hydration status. Delivering fluid via intravenous infusion or a gastric feeding tube allows researchers to bypass the oral receptors in the oral civility that would detect fluid and removes/reduces the requirement of the participants to drink.

Wall et al. (50) actively dehydrated individuals to 3% body mass losses (2 h exercise in the heat 33°C, 40% relative humidity) before restoring either 0%, 33%, or 100% of the fluid lost with the intravenous infusion of saline so that they were either 3%, 2%, or 0% hypohydrated. Following the rehydration phase, participants completed a 25 km cycling time trial in the heat (with realistic wind flow). Despite the large differences in hydration status, performance in this time trial did not differ between the three conditions and core temperature, skin temperature, heart rate, ratings of perceived exertion, thermal sensation, and thirst were also similar. The only difference was a higher core temperature from 17 km in the 3% hypohydration trial.

In a similar study, Cheung et al. (51) attempted to manipulate hydration and thirst. In order to do this, Cheung et al. (51) combined intravenous saline infusion with mouth rinsing. On four occasions, real or sham intravenous infusion was administered so that on two occasions participants were euhydrated (within ~0.5% of baseline body mass) and on two occasions participants were dehydrated (−2.5% of baseline body mass). During one of the euhydration trials and one of the hypohydration trials, participants were able to rinse their mouths with water to reduce the sensation of thirst. Similarly, to Wall et al. (50), hypohydration had no effect on power output during a 20 km time trial but interestingly neither did thirst. During the dehydration phase, heart rate and rectal temperatures were similar but they were higher during the time trial in both hypohydration conditions. Perceptual responses were similar.

Using a different approach, James et al. (52) used the gastric food tube method to investigate the effect of being hypohydrated on cycling performance. Seven healthy male cyclists undertook a 155 min sub-maximal (50%) cycling preload followed by a 15 min time trial in hot conditions (34°C, 50% RH) on two occasions. On both occasions, participants drank water (0.2 ml kg^{-1} every 10 min) with a feeding tube inserted to the base of the stomach. In the euhydration trial, participants had water infused at a rate to maintain euhydration, whilst in the other they did not. Infusing the water meant that participants finished the preload only ~0.1% different from when they started whereas in the other trial participants ended ~2.4% lighter. Hypohydrated participants ended the preload with higher heart rates, serum osmolality, arginine vasopressin concentrations, sensations of thirst, and ratings of perceived exertion but core body temperature and thermal sensations were similar between trials. Despite not knowing that hydration status had been manipulated, participants completed ~8% more work in the performance test when euhydrated compared to when hypohydrated.

These three studies have used two different ways to try to gain further insight into the role that hypohydration, and an individual's awareness of their hydration status, has on exercise performance and have reported opposing conclusions. Why? There are a number of reasons; these include:

Serum osmolality: James et al. (52) used water, which is hypotonic rather than isotonic, which meant that hyperosmolality was observed whereas it was not in the studies by Wall et al. (50) and Cheung et al. (51). This means that the hypohydration induced by James et al. is more physiologically similar to the hypohydration observed in the field.

Airflow: Realistic wind speed can reduce perceived and physiological strain, and so if it is lacking the effects of hypohydration may be exacerbated. James et al. (52) only had a very low level of convective cooling (~1 km·h^{-1}) whereas Wall et al. (50) and Cheung et al. (51) used more ecologically valid wind flow – ~32 km·h^{-1} and ~11 km·h^{-1}, respectively.

Thirst: By design, Cheung et al. (51) altered thirst sensations by allowing participants to rinse their mouths although thirst did not influence time-trial performance. Similar data were reported by Wall et al. (50) who reported similar thirst sensations despite not allowing participants to drink or mouth rinse although James et al. (52) observed higher sensations of thirst in the hypohydrated trial despite allowing for a small amount of fluid consumption.

8.5 Effects of hypohydration on cognitive performance in the heat

As discussed in Chapter 5, cognitive performance is an umbrella term for many functions or skills (e.g. attention, motor control, learning, memory, and reasoning), and can be assessed using a number of different tests. Due to the complex nature of cognitive function assessment, ascertaining the effects of hypohydration on cognitive performance is a challenge even in normal conditions. The challenge is even greater when exercise and hyperthermia are also present because during the early stages of exercise, activity may compensate for any hypohydration effect on cognitive function (53).

Body mass changes are most frequently used to quantify hydration status in cognitive function studies. It is often reported that hypohydration (1–3%) impairs cognitive function (54;55) and that the negative effect of hypohydration on cognitive function is proportionate to its magnitude i.e. you see greater impairments with greater levels of hypohydration (54); however, due to the complicated nature of cognitive performance, the effect of hypohydration appears more complicated than that. Hypohydration has no effect on reaction time (56;57), long-term memory (57), or perceptual task performance (57) but it slows down the decision-making processes (57) and impairs psychomotor tasks that require visuomotor or hand-to-eye coordination and short-term memory (57). Many of these impairments are reversible with rest and interestingly there may be no additional benefit to restoring cognitive performance by rehydrating compared to rest alone (57). It seems fair to say that some, but not all, aspects of cognitive performance are impaired by hypohydration but the mechanism(s) behind this are unclear. It has been suggested that impaired cognitive function in the heat may be due to hyperthermia-induced changes in blood–brain permeability and cerebral blood flow (58); however, 2% hypohydration would not raise plasma osmolality by enough to alter blood–brain permeability. Reductions in cerebral blood flow have been implicated but such reductions do not appear to result in reductions in cognitive function – in fact, exercise can improve cognitive function despite reductions in cerebral blood flow (59). Other theories suggest that impairment may only occur when athletes are thirsty (60) or when mood is impaired. Hypohydration sometimes (56;61–63), but not always (57), impairs mood state, and this may explain some of the impairment when it is observed; however, thirst and/or mood are not always measured during hypohydration-cognitive performance studies.

While the data regarding the effect of hypohydration on cognitive performance are mixed, there appears to be a consistent impairment on sport-specific performance. Sports performance involves a combination of athletic and cognitive performance and hypohydration can impair motor skill performance in a range of sports including cricket (64), basketball (65), golf (66), and field hockey (67). Macleod and Sunderland (67) reported that elite female hockey players' hockey-specific performance and decision-making time were impaired when they were ~2% hypohydrated. The players were required to complete a field hockey-specific skills test and took longer to do so when hypohydrated because they incurred time penalties for errors made (i.e. kicking the ball, touching a cone, missing the target). When looking to optimise athletic performance, stand-alone cognitive tests offer some insight into the effects of hypohydration; however, more ecologically valid tests should be adopted. While it appears that the effect of hypohydration on cognitive performance is mixed, the negative effect on complex sport-specific skills performance appears less contentious.

8.6 Exercise-associated hyponatremia (EAH)

Hyponatremia describes a medical condition in which an athlete has a very low extracellular sodium concentration (less than 135 mmol·L^{-1}) (2). Typical symptoms of hyponatremia include headaches, vomiting, and altered mental statement but most athletes suffering from hyponatremia will be asymptomatic (i.e. they will not display any signs of hyponatremia and can only be diagnosed by analysing post-exercise blood samples). The incidence of symptomatic hyponatremia (≤1%) is much lower than the incidence of asymptomatic hyponatremia (6–13%) (68;69); however, due to the need for blood analysis to confirm asymptomatic hyponatremia, the actual incidence is unknown in most settings. The most common and concerning form of hyponatremia is dilutional hyponatremia caused by the overconsumption of fluids and an arginine vasopressin-regulated reduction in water excretion. The main risk factors for dilutional hyponatremia are anything that might facilitate the overconsumption of fluid relative to sweat loss, e.g.

- Exercise duration >4 h
- Novice athlete
- High frequency of opportunities to drink, e.g. water stations too close together
- Slow running pace
- High or low body mass index

Many elite athletes will be unable to overconsume fluids due the nature of their sport (slower runners tend to have more opportunities to drink and are therefore at a greater risk of developing hyponatremia) but hyponatremia does affect elite athletes when there are sufficient opportunities to overconsume (e.g. American football). The most effective way to prevent hyponatremia is to educate athletes about the risk of overconsumption and to change drinking behaviour where required (22). For healthy athletes, drinking to thirst will prevent hyponatremia in most cases (22).

If overdrinking does occur and hyponatremia develops, efficient and accurate diagnosis and treatment is required because hyponatremia can be fatal. Asymptomatic hyponatremia can be treated by restricting hypotonic and isotonic fluid provision and administering hypertonic saline solution in order to prevent the potential progression from asymptomatic hyponatremia to symptomatic hyponatremia (70). Severe symptomatic hyponatremia is a potentially life-threatening situation that requires the immediate infusion of hypertonic saline solution (71;72) with additional boluses administered until there is clinical improvement (71;72). Less severe hyponatremia can be treated with intravenous or oral hypertonic fluid (70).

8.7 Hydration strategies

This section will help you with Problem 8.2: "Optimising hydration for the team-sport athlete": "You are a sport scientist working for a semi-professional football club. You have a busy pre-season period coming up and the weather is going to be warm (28–35°C). What hydration strategies can you adopt? Why?"

When devising a hydration strategy, a number of things merit consideration. These include:

- Environmental conditions
- Individual preferences
- Frequency of drinking opportunities
- Individual familiarisation with a hypohydrated state
- Acclimation/acclimatisation state

8.7.1 Pre-exercise

Athletes often start exercise hypohydrated (73) and so a pre-exercise fluid regimen may be required. It has been suggested that athletes should drink sufficient fluids to produce urine that is either very pale, or pale, yellow (20), and to keep the sensation of thirst as low as possible prior to exercise (74). It is recommended that athletes drink 500–600 ml 2–3 h before an event followed by 200–300 ml 10–20 min before the start of the event (75). Drinking fluids containing sodium before exercise can help with fluid retention and subsequently establishing a state of euhydration (24)

8.7.2 Per-exercise

Gastric emptying rate is reduced during higher intensity exercise (76) and so it is difficult to replace fluid lost during exercise. Whilst cycling, consuming fluid at a rate of $0.15-0.34$ ml·kg^{-1}·min^{-1} reduces power output by ~2.5% during 1 h of high intensity (>80% peak oxygen consumption) exercise compared to no fluid consumption whereas intakes of $0.14-0.27$ ml·kg^{-1}·min^{-1} during exercise are associated with improved cycling performance in 20–33°C temperatures (77). Cycling is one sport where fluid availability is relatively high, but drinking during many other sports is more difficult. Maughan et al. (78) reported that during a preseason training session in warm conditions (24°C–29°C), English Premier League soccer players lost 2.0 ± 0.4 L of sweat (range: 1.3–2.8 L) but only drank 971 ± 331 ml (range: 265–1,661 ml) resulting in mean body mass loss of ~1.4%. There were large individual variations, meaning that while some soccer players ended the session hypohydrated (body mass loss of 2.6%), others were marginally so (0.45% body mass loss). The fluid consumptions reported by Maughan et al. (78) were higher than those often observed in team sports (79), and the authors suggested that this might have been due to the warm conditions and/ or the fact that the participants knew that they were expected to provide data regarding their hydration status and practices. Athletes in hot conditions will typically end the session or event hypohydrated and so interventions should be put in place to facilitate fluid consumption where possible e.g. providing the beverages at a palatable temperature; however, caution should be taken to prevent overconsumption.

8.7.3 Post-exercise

Structured rehydration strategies are usually only required if there is less than 4 h between exercise bouts or if body mass losses in excess of 5% are observed (16;24); however, athlete urine samples collected pre-exercise frequently display hyperosmolality indicating that athletes frequently commence exercise in a hypohydrated state (78). Quickly drinking large volumes of hypotonic fluid can result in an increase in blood volume and a reduction in plasma osmolality and arginine vasopressin release (80), and so athletes should avoid drinking too quickly post-exercise. Replacing fluids at a volume of 100% of what was lost is more effective over a 240 min period compared to a 60 min one (81) but although the rehydration rate was greater in the longer duration trial, participants did not reach euhydration in either. In order to reach euhydration, a volume in excess of the amount lost is required in the hour following exercise to restore a state of euhydration (17). Drinking 150% of the volume lost is more effective at restoring euhydration status than ingesting 100% of the volume lost when ingested over a period of 60 (17) and 180 min (82) following exercise.

Ingesting plain water should be avoided because doing so can cause large reductions in plasma sodium concentration and osmolality (83) and the excretion, rather than retention, of the fluid ingested. To prevent this, the fluid should have a relatively large sodium content to facilitate rehydration (17). For example, during the first 60 min following exercise, net fluid gain can be similar between plain water and water containing 0.45% of sodium chloride but plasma volume restoration is greater (60% versus 17%), and plasma osmolality is elevated for longer, when the water is supplemented with sodium chloride (83). Sports drinks tend to have a sodium concentration of ~20 mmol·L^{-1} which seems to be effective at improving rehydration (Shirreffs et al. (17) reported effective rehydration with 23 mmol·L^{-1}) but 200% replacement may offer further benefit if the sodium concentration is increased to 61 mmol·L^{-1} (17).

8.7.4 Prescribed versus "to thirst"

The American College of Sports Medicine revised its recommendations in 2007. Until 2006, the recommendations were that athletes should "consume fluids at a rate sufficient to replace the water lost through sweating or consume the maximum amount that can be tolerated" (84). Current recommendations are that athletes should adopt an individualised fluid intake program that minimises body mass loss to <2% (24). There is a lot of debate regarding whether drinking to thirst is an appropriate drinking strategy. Hoffman and colleagues (85;86) and Armstrong et al. (87;88) participated in a point-counterpoint discussion and the main viewpoints are summarised in Table 8.3.

TABLE 8.3 Summary of point-counterpoint discussion between Hoffman and colleagues (85;86) and Armstrong et al. (87;88)

Drinking to thirst is adequate to maintain hydration status during prolonged endurance exercise (85;86)	Drinking to thirst is NOT adequate to maintain hydration status during prolonged endurance exercise (87;88)
Increased risk of hyponatremia	Data are lacking regarding the effectiveness of drinking to thirst in the prevention of hyponatremia
Due to water storage, body mass loss does not necessarily indicate hypohydration	Thirst can be satiated quickly upon drinking
Hypohydration <4% does not impair real-world exercise performance	Hypohydration ~1.5% can impair strength, power, and endurance exercise
Recommendations are often made from poorly designed studies e.g. those without realistic head-wind and/or blinding	This is somewhat offset by the lack of solar radiation. It is often difficult to confirm the role of thirst in the studies which show no effect of hypohydration
Body mass losses >2% are well tolerated by elite athletes	Hypohydration can increase physiological strain in athletes
Prescribed drinking can cause gastrointestinal distress	Optimal hydration strategies are individual- and situational-specific and may include thirst
Prescribing fluid based upon estimated sweat loss data lacks accuracy	Individualised plans can be designed based upon multiple data sets Drinking to thirst may be inappropriate for heavy sweaters
Drinking to thirst and ad libitum fluid consumption appear to have similar results during exercise when athletes have adequate access to fluid	Drinking to thirst is not the same as drinking ad libitum Drinking to thirst is an instruction that can be interpreted in a number of ways
Drinking to thirst is an evolutionary adaptation to survival	Evolutionary adaptations have no relevance to modern-day sporting events because they were not selective pressures
Thirst may be initiated at hypohydration <1%	Thirst is only initiated when body mass loss reach ~2%

Problem 8.1 revisited: Assessment of hydration status in the field

You are a sports scientist working for a local athletics club and wish to begin a programme of hydration monitoring with your athletes. You have a budget of £200 for this and see each athlete twice a week. Which method, or methods, would you use? Why?

The gold standard is plasma osmolality; however, this requires expensive equipment and so with a budget of only £200 measuring the osmolality of any fluid (plasma or urine) is out of the question.

USG is a possibility although refractometers tend to be more expensive than £200. You might be able to find a cheap refractometer to measure USG and if you can this approach is advised because this measure has a moderate relationship with plasma osmolality (18) and urine osmolality (19). Be wary, though, because USG can underestimate hydration status.

Urine colour assessed using the scale devised by Armstrong et al. (20) is well correlated with urine osmolality and USG and so is an acceptable form of assessment in many applied settings. Maintaining urine that is "very pale yellow", "pale yellow", or "straw-coloured" is likely to be a good indicator of euhydration; however, urine colour should not be used when precise and accurate data are required. The scale is widely available but do take care to ensure that the correct colours are printed.

What about nude body mass change? A first morning, post-urination, body mass will vary by less than 1% for a well-hydrated athlete in energy balance (23;24) and so it is a cheap, easy way to estimate hydration status on a day-to-day basis. Scales should be calibrated and measurements should be made on at least three consecutive days to establish a baseline value from which to evaluate deviations (23). If you are assessing female athletes, remember to standardise the phase of the menstrual cycle at which measurements are taken.

Although cheap and relatively quick, clinical assessment markers are unable to detect body mass losses of >3% (28) and so they should not be used.

Summary: While osmolality would be ideal, your budget does not stretch to using it. If you can pick up a cheap refractometer USG would be a good measurement to take; however, you might be reliant on body mass changes and urine colour. These two assessment techniques are inexpensive and easy to administer and can easily be run together as part of a hydration assessment approach.

Problem 8.2 revisited: Optimising hydration for the team sport athlete

You are a sports scientist working for a semi-professional football club. You have a busy pre-season period coming up and the weather is going to be warm (28–35°C). What hydration strategies should you adopt?

We do not know the acclimation state or individual preferences of the players (although in a real-world scenario you might) but we do know that the conditions are going to be hot and that football matches offer good opportunities for fluid consumption before, at half-time, and at the end, but that opportunities during the match itself are limited.

- Providing drinks at a palatable temperature (usually 10–15°C is preferred)
- Ensuring that drinks are available. Some sports have sufficient breaks in play to enable athletes to take on fluid, but others do not, and so coaches and support staff should consider how to get fluids to their players during periods of play.
- Not adding too much sugar to beverages as doing so can decrease acceptability. Trained athletes reported that glucose-electrolyte drinks containing 12% glucose caused significantly more nausea and fullness than either 6% glucose or water and so were less likely to choose the more concentrated drink during training or competition (89).
- Sodium is required to ensure the maintenance of the extracellular fluid volume. Humans have a specific appetite for salt (sodium chloride), but, despite possessing an appetite for salt, athletes who lose a lot salt through sweating do not have an appetite sufficient to replace the salt lost (1). Salt should be added to the fluid consumed when sweat losses are high (3–4 g of sodium) and during prolonged (>2 h) exercise (90).

8.8 Summary

Humans are ~60% water and so deviations in hydration status can have implications for many things including health, mood, and exercise performance. Measuring hydration status is easy to do but difficult to do well. Plasma osmolality is considered the "gold standard" approach to hydration assessment with euhydration defined as an osmolality of 280–290 mOsmol (1). Plasma osmolality is an invasive technique that requires the drawing of blood and so midstream urinary osmolality is sometimes used with a euhydration cut-off of <700 mOsmol. Other ways to measure hydration status (e.g. USG, urine colour, body mass changes) can be used; however, they are all less direct and as a result less accurate.

Hydration status fluctuates between states of hyper- and hypo-hydration and it has been proposed that hypohydrated states should be avoided as an athlete. Hypohydration decreases whole-body sweating (29) and increases the threshold for sweat onset, resulting in a typical increase in core body temperature of approximately 0.1–0.2°C for every 1% hypohydration (30). Hypohydration decreases plasma volume and as a result elevates heart rate and total peripheral resistance while decreasing blood volume, mean arterial pressure, stroke volume, cardiac output, limb blood flow, skin blood flow, and cerebral blood flow (31). These (and other) physiological responses can have an impact on cognitive and exercise performance with Sawka et al. (39) reporting regular impairments in the ability to exercise in hot conditions (>25°C; 8/9 studies) and occasional impairments in temperate conditions (20–24°C; 4/7 studies). The effect of hypo-hydration on exercise performance is a somewhat contentious topic with many researchers pointing to the fact that elite athletes are often severely hypohydrated at the end of prolonged sporting events. Despite the controversy, meta-analysis data suggest that muscle endurance, strength, and anaerobic power are all im-paired by hypohydration (41). Dehydration, hypohydration, and thirst are often researched together but researchers have sought to separate the effects of thirst from hypohydration. Thirst is defined as a desire to drink due to a deficit of water (increases in plasma osmolality is the primary driver for the thirst response) and some researchers have demonstrated that exercise performance is unaffected if an individual is hypohydrated but not thirsty. This topic requires further research.

Despite the controversy, hydration strategies are often adopted by athletes and they should be specific to the sport (e.g. when is drinking possible?), athlete (what are their personal preferences?), and environmental conditions (is it hot?). Athletes often start exercise hypohydrated (73) and so it is recommended that athletes consume sufficient fluid prior to completion to produce urine that is either very pale, or pale, yellow (20), and to keep the sensation of thirst as low as possible prior to exercise (74). Fluid consumption during exercise can be dif-ficult (especially during high-intensity exercise) due to a reduction in the gas-tric emptying rate (76), and so athletes often lose more fluid than they replace. As a result, usually the best time to restore hydration status is after the event; however, structured rehydration strategies are usually only required if there is less than 4 h between exercise bouts or if body mass losses in excess of 5% are observed (16;24). If a structured strategy is required, athletes should drink a volume equivalent to ~150% of what was lost over a period of 1–3 h and the fluid consumed should have a sodium concentration of ~20 mmol·L^{-1} to prevent large reductions in plasma osmolality (83) and facilitate fluid retention. The overconsumption of fluids (especially those without added sodium) can result in EAH, and so care should be taken not to overprescribe fluids. In elite settings, the opportunities to drink are often limited which reduces the risk but if EAH does occur, efficient and accurate diagnosis and treatment is required because hyponatremia can be fatal.

8.9 Self-check quiz

At the beginning of this chapter you were told that by this point you should know the answers to the following broad questions:

- Why is maintaining hydration status important for an athlete?
- Does hydration status influence exercise performance?
- How can you assess hydration status and what is the best approach?
- What are the physiological responses to hypohydration?
- Are there any risks to over-hydrating?

In order to see whether you do now know the answers to these questions, have a go at this short self-check quiz. The answers follow the questions, but before looking at the answers, if you are stuck on any question, try looking back at the relevant section. For help with questions 1–4, take another look at Section 8.1; the answers to questions 5–7 can be found in Section 8.2; the answer to question 8 can be found in Section 8.3; and the answers to questions 9 and 10 can be found in Section 8.5.

8.9.1 Self-check quiz questions

1. Approximately how much (as a percentage) of the human body is made up of water?
2. Is most of the body's water contained in the intra- or extra-cellular compartments?
3. What is the difference between "hypohydration" and "dehydration"?
4. In what two main ways is thirst triggered?
5. What is considered the "gold standard" of hydration assessment?
6. When using the gold standard method (see question 5!), what is the range considered "euhydration"?
7. What does urine specific gravity measure?
8. When hypohydrated, what happens to core body temperature and heart rate?
9. What is exercise associated hyponatremia and what causes it?
10. What are the five main risk factors for exercise-associated hyponatremia?

8.9.2 Self-check quiz answers

1. ~60% (but can range from as little as 45% to as much as 75%).
2. Intracellular (~65% of the total body water).
3. Hypohydration describes a state where body masses are lower than normal whereas dehydration describes the process of losing water.
4. Increased arginine vasopressin which is released in response to increased osmolality (detected by osmoreceptors) and 2) decreased blood volume (detected by baroreceptors).
5. Plasma osmolality.
6. Euhydration is defined as a plasma osmolality of 280–290 mOsmol.
7. The density of urine compared to the density of water. It normally ranges between 1.003 and 1.035 with euhydrated often being defined as a USG value of between 1.010 and 1.020.
8. Both increase compared to euhydrated values.
9. Hyponatremia is a reduction in the sodium concentration within the extracellular fluid (*hypo* (low) + *natrium* (sodium)) caused by the overconsumption of hypotonic fluids (e.g. water).
10. The five main risk factors for exercise-associated hyponatremia are:

1   An exercise duration >4 h
2   A novice athlete
3   A high frequency of opportunities to drink e.g. water stations too close together
4   A slow running pace
5   A high or low body mass index

8.10 Practical toolkit

TOOLBOX 8.1 QUICK REFERENCE TABLE – HYDRATION STRATEGIES

Remember that when you are devising a hydration strategy you need to consider the environmental conditions, individual preferences, the frequency of drinking opportunities, the athlete's familiarisation with a hypohydrated state, and the heat acclimation/acclimatisation status of the athlete (Table 8.4).

TABLE 8.4 Quick reference – hydration strategies

	Aim	Recommendation(s)
Pre-exercise	The athlete commences exercise in an optimal hydration state	1. 500–600 ml 2–3 h before an event 2. 200–300 ml 10–20 min before the start of the event 3. Sodium can be added to the fluid to aid fluid retention 4. Drink sufficient fluids to produce urine that is either very pale, or pale, yellow
Per-exercise	Minimise fluid losses Maintain athlete's preferred hydration and thirst status	1. Ensure that fluids are available 2. Consider introducing drink breaks 3. Encourage athletes to drink to regulate thirst
Post-exercise	Restore fluid lost during exercise	1. Have a structured rehydration strategy if there is less than without 4 h between bouts and body mass losses exceed 5% 2. Drink slowly to maintain arginine vasopressin release 3. Drink ~150% of body mass losses over 60–180 min 4. Avoid drinking plain water – add ~20 mmol.L−1 of sodium to the drink

TOOLBOX 8.2 ESTIMATING SWEAT LOSS AND RATE

It is easy to estimate sweat rate using only a set of weighing scales. Figure 8.1 shows you how.

	Body mass before exercise (kg)	Body mass after exercise (kg)	Mass of the full water bottles before exercise (kg or l)	Mass of the water bottles after exercise (kg or l)	Urine loss while exercising (kg or l)	Exercise duration (hours)
	A	B	C	D	E	F
Example	64.50	63.70	0.500	0.370	0.00	2

			Example data	Answer
Sweat loss (l) =	total non-urinary fluid lost during exercise	= (A − B) - E	(64.50 − 63.70) - 0.00	0.800
	+			+
	total fluid consumed during exercise	= C − D	0.500 − 0.370	0.130
				0.930
Sweat rate (l·min⁻¹) =	sweat loss / exercise duration	= 0.930 / F	0.930 / 2	0.465

FIGURE 8.1 Estimating sweat loss and rate.

References

1 Senay LC, Jr. Temperature regulation and hypohydration: a singular view. *J Appl Physiol Respir Environ Exerc Physiol* 1979 Jul;47(1):1–7.

2 McDermott BP, Anderson SA, Armstrong LE, Casa DJ, Cheuvront SN, Cooper L, et al. National Athletic Trainers' Association position statement: fluid replacement for the physically active. *J Athl Train* 2017 Sep;52(9):877–95.

3 Greenleaf JE. Problem: thirst, drinking behavior, and involuntary dehydration. *Med Sci Sports Exerc* 1992 Jun;24(6):645–56.

4 Verbalis JG. Disorders of body water homeostasis. *Best Pract Res Clin Endocrinol Metab* 2003 Dec;17(4):471–503.

5 Baylis PH, Robertson GL. Plasma vasopressin response to hypertonic saline infusion to assess posterior pituitary function. *J R Soc Med* 1980 Apr;73(4):255–60.

6 Zerbe RL, Miller JZ, Robertson GL. The reproducibility and heritability of individual differences in osmoregulatory function in normal human subjects. *J Lab Clin Med* 1991 Jan;117(1):51–9.

7 McKenna K, Thompson C. Osmoregulation in clinical disorders of thirst appreciation. *Clin Endocrinol (Oxf)* 1998 Aug;49(2):139–52.

8 Thompson CJ, Burd JM, Baylis PH. Acute suppression of plasma vasopressin and thirst after drinking in hypernatremic humans. *Am J Physiol* 1987 Jun;252(6 Pt 2): R1138–R1142.

9 Bourque CW. Central mechanisms of osmosensation and systemic osmoregulation. *Nat Rev Neurosci* 2008 Jul;9(7):519–31.

10 Denton D, Shade R, Zamarippa F, Egan G, Blair-West J, McKinley M, et al. Correlation of regional cerebral blood flow and change of plasma sodium concentration during genesis and satiation of thirst. *Proc Natl Acad Sci U S A* 1999 Mar 2;96(5):2532–7.

11 Geelen G, Keil LC, Kravik SE, Wade CE, Thrasher TN, Barnes PR, et al. Inhibition of plasma vasopressin after drinking in dehydrated humans. *Am J Physiol* 1984 Dec;247(6 Pt 2):R968–R971.

12 Rolls BJ, Wood RJ, Rolls ET, Lind H, Lind W, Ledingham JG. Thirst following water deprivation in humans. *Am J Physiol* 1980 Nov;239(5):R476–R482.

13 Phillips S, Hutchinson S, Davidson T. Preoperative drinking does not affect gastric contents. *Br J Anaesth* 1993 Jan;70(1):6–9.

14 Engell DB, Maller O, Sawka MN, Francesconi RN, Drolet L, Young AJ. Thirst and fluid intake following graded hypohydration levels in humans. *Physiol Behav* 1987;40(2):229–36.

15 Cheuvront SN, Ely BR, Kenefick RW, Sawka MN. Biological variation and diagnostic accuracy of dehydration assessment markers. *Am J Clin Nutr* 2010 Sep;92(3):565–73.

16 Shirreffs SM, Sawka MN. Fluid and electrolyte needs for training, competition, and recovery. *J Sports Sci* 2011;29 Suppl 1:S39–S46.

17 Shirreffs SM, Taylor AJ, Leiper JB, Maughan RJ. Post-exercise rehydration in man: effects of volume consumed and drink sodium content. *Med Sci Sports Exerc* 1996 Oct;28(10):1260–71.

18 Popowski LA, Oppliger RA, Patrick LG, Johnson RF, Kim JA, Gisolf CV. Blood and urinary measures of hydration status during progressive acute dehydration. *Med Sci Sports Exerc* 2001 May;33(5):747–53.

19 Hew-Butler TD, Eskin C, Bickham J, Rusnak M, VanderMeulen M. Dehydration is how you define it: comparison of 318 blood and urine athlete spot checks. *BMJ Open Sport Exerc Med* 2018;4(1):e000297.

20 Armstrong LE, Maresh CM, Castellani JW, Bergeron MF, Kenefick RW, LaGasse KE, et al. Urinary indices of hydration status. *Int J Sport Nutr* 1994 Sep;4(3):265–79.

21 McKenzie AL, Munoz CX, Armstrong LE. Accuracy of urine color to detect equal to or greater than 2% body mass loss in men. *J Athl Train* 2015 Dec;50(12):1306–9.

22 Hew-Butler T, Rosner MH, Fowkes-Godek S, Dugas JP, Hoffman MD, Lewis DP, et al. Statement of the 3rd International Exercise-Associated Hyponatremia Consensus Development Conference, Carlsbad, California, 2015. *Br J Sports Med* 2015 Nov;49(22):1432–46.

23 Cheuvront SN, Carter R, III, Montain SJ, Sawka MN. Daily body mass variability and stability in active men undergoing exercise-heat stress. *Int J Sport Nutr Exerc Metab* 2004 Oct;14(5):532–40.

24 Sawka MN, Burke LM, Eichner ER, Maughan RJ, Montain SJ, Stachenfeld NS. American College of Sports Medicine position stand. Exercise and fluid replacement. *Med Sci Sports Exerc* 2007 Feb;39(2):377–90.

25 Bunt JC, Lohman TG, Boileau RA. Impact of total body water fluctuations on estimation of body fat from body density. *Med Sci Sports Exerc* 1989 Feb;21(1):96–100.

26 Cheuvront SN, Haymes EM, Sawka MN. Comparison of sweat loss estimates for women during prolonged high-intensity running. *Med Sci Sports Exerc* 2002 Aug;34(8):1344–50.

27 Mitchell JW, Nadel ER, Stolwijk JA. Respiratory weight losses during exercise. *J Appl Physiol* 1972 Apr;32(4):474–6.

28 McGarvey J, Thompson J, Hanna C, Noakes TD, Stewart J, Speedy D. Sensitivity and specificity of clinical signs for assessment of dehydration in endurance athletes. *Br J Sports Med* 2010 Aug;44(10):716–9.

29 Sawka MN, Young AJ, Francesconi RP, Muza SR, Pandolf KB. Thermoregulatory and blood responses during exercise at graded hypohydration levels. *J Appl Physiol (1985)* 1985 Nov;59(5):1394–401.

30 Sawka MN, Francesconi RP, Young AJ, Pandolf KB. Influence of hydration level and body fluids on exercise performance in the heat. *JAMA* 1984 Sep 7;252(9):1165–9.

31 Trangmar SJ, Gonzalez-Alonso J. New insights into the impact of dehydration on blood flow and metabolism during exercise. *Exerc Sport Sci Rev* 2017 Jul;45(3):146–53.

32 Costill DL, Cote R, Fink W. Muscle water and electrolytes following varied levels of dehydration in man. *J Appl Physiol* 1976 Jan;40(1):6–11.

33 Stohr EJ, Gonzalez-Alonso J, Pearson J, Low DA, Ali L, Barker H, et al. Dehydration reduces left ventricular filling at rest and during exercise independent of twist mechanics. *J Appl Physiol (1985)* 2011 Sep;111(3):891–7.

34 Gonzalez-Alonso J, Mora-Rodriguez R, Below PR, Coyle EF. Dehydration reduces cardiac output and increases systemic and cutaneous vascular resistance during exercise. *J Appl Physiol (1985)* 1995 Nov;79(5):1487–96.

35 Gonzalez-Alonso J, Mora-Rodriguez R, Below PR, Coyle EF. Dehydration markedly impairs cardiovascular function in hyperthermic endurance athletes during exercise. *J Appl Physiol (1985)* 1997 Apr;82(4):1229–36.

36 Segar WE, Moore WW. The regulation of antidiuretic hormone release in man: I. Effects of change in position and ambient temperature on blood ADH levels. *J Clin Invest* 1968 Sep;47(9):2143–51.

37 Nose H, Mack GW, Shi XR, Nadel ER. Involvement of sodium retention hormones during rehydration in humans. *J Appl Physiol (1985)* 1988 Jul;65(1):332–6.

38 Sawka MN, Cheuvront SN, Kenefick RW. High skin temperature and hypohydration impair aerobic performance. *Exp Physiol* 2012 Mar;97(3):327–32.

39 Sawka MN, Cheuvront SN, Kenefick RW. Hypohydration and human performance: impact of environment and physiological mechanisms. *Sports Med* 2015 Nov;45(Suppl 1):S51–S60.

40 Cheuvront SN, Kenefick RW. Dehydration: physiology, assessment, and performance effects. *Compr Physiol* 2014 Jan;4(1):257–85.

41 Savoie FA, Kenefick RW, Ely BR, Cheuvront SN, Goulet ED. Effect of hypohydration on muscle endurance, strength, anaerobic power and capacity and vertical jumping ability: a meta-analysis. *Sports Med* 2015 Aug;45(8):1207–27.

42 Goulet ED. Effect of exercise-induced dehydration on time-trial exercise performance: a meta-analysis. *Br J Sports Med* 2011 Nov;45(14):1149–56.

43 Cheuvront SN, Montain SJ, Sawka MN. Fluid replacement and performance during the marathon. *Sports Med* 2007;37(4–5):353–7.

44 Zouhal H, Groussard C, Minter G, Vincent S, Cretual A, Gratas-Delamarche A, et al. Inverse relationship between percentage body weight change and finishing time in 643 forty-two-kilometre marathon runners. *Br J Sports Med* 2011 Nov;45(14):1101–5.

45 Sharwood KA, Collins M, Goedecke JH, Wilson G, Noakes TD. Weight changes, medical complications, and performance during an Ironman triathlon. *Br J Sports Med* 2004 Dec;38(6):718–24.

46 Kao WF, Shyu CL, Yang XW, Hsu TF, Chen JJ, Kao WC, et al. Athletic performance and serial weight changes during 12- and 24-hour ultra-marathons. *Clin J Sport Med* 2008 Mar;18(2):155–8.

47 Pugh LG, Corbett JL, Johnson RH. Rectal temperatures, weight losses, and sweat rates in marathon running. *J Appl Physiol* 1967 Sep;23(3):347–52.

48 Beis LY, Wright-Whyte M, Fudge B, Noakes T, Pitsiladis YP. Drinking behaviors of elite male runners during marathon competition. *Clin J Sport Med* 2012 May;22(3):254–61.

49 Fleming J, James LJ. Repeated familiarisation with hypohydration attenuates the performance decrement caused by hypohydration during treadmill running. *Appl Physiol Nutr Metab* 2014 Feb;39(2):124–9.

50 Wall BA, Watson G, Peiffer JJ, Abbiss CR, Siegel R, Laursen PB. Current hydration guidelines are erroneous: dehydration does not impair exercise performance in the heat. *Br J Sports Med* 2015 Aug;49(16):1077–83.

51 Cheung SS, McGarr GW, Mallette MM, Wallace PJ, Watson CL, Kim IM, et al. Separate and combined effects of dehydration and thirst sensation on exercise performance in the heat. *Scand J Med Sci Sports* 2015 Jun;25(Suppl 1):104–11.

52 James LJ, Moss J, Henry J, Papadopoulou C, Mears SA. Hypohydration impairs endurance performance: a blinded study. *Physiol Rep* 2017 Jun;5(12):e13315.

53 Maughan RJ, Shirreffs SM, Watson P. Exercise, heat, hydration and the brain. *J Am Coll Nutr* 2007 Oct;26(5 Suppl):604S–12S.

54 Gopinathan PM, Pichan G, Sharma VM. Role of dehydration in heat stress-induced variations in mental performance. *Arch Environ Health* 1988 Jan;43(1):15–7.

55 Lindseth PD, Lindseth GN, Petros TV, Jensen WC, Caspers J. Effects of hydration on cognitive function of pilots. *Mil Med* 2013 Jul;178(7):792–8.

56 D'anci KE, Vibhakar A, Kanter JH, Mahoney CR, Taylor HA. Voluntary dehydration and cognitive performance in trained college athletes. *Percept Mot Skills* 2009 Aug;109(1):251–69.

57 Cian C, Barraud PA, Melin B, Raphel C. Effects of fluid ingestion on cognitive function after heat stress or exercise-induced dehydration. *Int J Psychophysiol* 2001 Nov;42(3):243–51.

58 Nybo L, Moller K, Volianitis S, Nielsen B, Secher NH. Effects of hyperthermia on cerebral blood flow and metabolism during prolonged exercise in humans. *J Appl Physiol* 2002 Jul;93(1):58–64.

59 Ogoh S, Tsukamoto H, Hirasawa A, Hasegawa H, Hirose N, Hashimoto T. The effect of changes in cerebral blood flow on cognitive function during exercise. *Physiol Rep* 2014 Sep 1;2(9):e12163.

60 Edmonds CJ, Crombie R, Gardner MR. Subjective thirst moderates changes in speed of responding associated with water consumption. *Front Hum Neurosci* 2013;7:363.

61 Armstrong LE, Ganio MS, Casa DJ, Lee EC, McDermott BP, Klau JF, et al. Mild dehydration affects mood in healthy young women. *J Nutr* 2012 Feb;142(2):382–8.

62 Ganio MS, Armstrong LE, Casa DJ, McDermott BP, Lee EC, Yamamoto LM, et al. Mild dehydration impairs cognitive performance and mood of men. *Br J Nutr* 2011 Nov;106(10):1535–43.

63 Moyen NE, Ganio MS, Wiersma LD, Kavouras SA, Gray M, McDermott BP, et al. Hydration status affects mood state and pain sensation during ultra-endurance cycling. *J Sports Sci* 2015;33(18):1962–9.

64 Gamage JP, De Silva AP, Nalliah AK, Galloway SD. Effects of dehydration on cricket specific skill performance in hot and humid conditions. *Int J Sport Nutr Exerc Metab* 2016 Dec;26(6):531–41.

65 Baker LB, Dougherty KA, Chow M, Kenney WL. Progressive dehydration causes a progressive decline in basketball skill performance. *Med Sci Sports Exerc* 2007 Jul;39(7):1114–23.

66 Smith MF, Newell AJ, Baker MR. Effect of acute mild dehydration on cognitive-motor performance in golf. *J Strength Cond Res* 2012 Nov;26(11):3075–80.

67 Macleod H, Sunderland C. Previous-day hypohydration impairs skill performance in elite female field hockey players. *Scand J Med Sci Sports* 2012 Jun;22(3):430–8.

68 Hoffman MD, Hew-Butler T, Stuempfle KJ. Exercise-associated hyponatremia and hydration status in 161-km ultramarathoners. *Med Sci Sports Exerc* 2013 Apr;45(4):784–91.

69 Noakes TD, Sharwood K, Speedy D, Hew T, Reid S, Dugas J, et al. Three independent biological mechanisms cause exercise-associated hyponatremia: evidence from 2,135 weighed competitive athletic performances. *Proc Natl Acad Sci U S A* 2005 Dec 20;102(51):18550–5.

70 Owen BE, Rogers IR, Hoffman MD, Stuempfle KJ, Lewis D, Fogard K, et al. Efficacy of oral versus intravenous hypertonic saline in runners with hyponatremia. *J Sci Med Sport* 2014 Sep;17(5):457–62.

71 Elsaesser TF, Pang PS, Malik S, Chiampas GT. Large-volume hypertonic saline therapy in endurance athlete with exercise-associated hyponatremic encephalopathy. *J Emerg Med* 2013 Jun;44(6):1132–5.

72 Hoffman MD, Stuempfle KJ, Sullivan K, Weiss RH. Exercise-associated hyponatremia with exertional rhabdomyolysis: importance of proper treatment. *Clin Nephrol* 2015 Apr;83(4):235–42.

73 Maughan RJ, Watson P, Evans GH, Broad N, Shirreffs SM. Water balance and salt losses in competitive football. *Int J Sport Nutr Exerc Metab* 2007 Dec;17(6):583–94.

74 Casa DJ, Stearns RL, Lopez RM, Ganio MS, McDermott BP, Walker YS, et al. Influence of hydration on physiological function and performance during trail running in the heat. *J Athl Train* 2010 Mar;45(2):147–56.

75 Casa DJ, Armstrong LE, Hillman SK, Montain SJ, Reiff RV, Rich BS, et al. National Athletic Trainers Association's position statement: fluid replacement for athletes. *J Athl Train* 2000 Apr;35(2):212–24.

76 Costill DL, Saltin B. Factors limiting gastric emptying during rest and exercise. *J Appl Physiol* 1974 Nov;37(5):679–83.

77 Holland JJ, Skinner TL, Irwin CG, Leveritt MD, Goulet EDB. The influence of drinking fluid on endurance cycling performance: a meta-analysis. *Sports Med* 2017 Nov;47(11):2269–84.

78 Maughan RJ, Merson SJ, Broad NP, Shirreffs SM. Fluid and electrolyte intake and loss in elite soccer players during training. *Int J Sport Nutr Exerc Metab* 2004 Jun;14(3):333–46.

79 Burke LM, Hawley JA. Fluid balance in team sports. Guidelines for optimal practices. *Sports Med* 1997 Jul;24(1):38–54.

80 Robertson GL. Vasopressin in osmotic regulation in man. *Annu Rev Med* 1974;25:315–22.

81 Jones EJ, Bishop PA, Green JM, Richardson MT. Effects of metered versus bolus water consumption on urine production and rehydration. *Int J Sport Nutr Exerc Metab* 2010 Apr;20(2):139–44.

82 Mitchell JB, Grandjean PW, Pizza FX, Starling RD, Holtz RW. The effect of volume ingested on rehydration and gastric emptying following exercise-induced dehydration. *Med Sci Sports Exerc* 1994 Sep;26(9):1135–43.

83 Nose H, Mack GW, Shi XR, Nadel ER. Role of osmolality and plasma volume during rehydration in humans. *J Appl Physiol (1985)* 1988 Jul;65(1):325–31.

84 Convertino VA, Armstrong LE, Coyle EF, Mack GW, Sawka MN, Senay LC, Jr., et al. American College of Sports Medicine position stand. Exercise and fluid replacement. *Med Sci Sports Exerc* 1996 Jan;28(1):i–vii.

85 Hoffman MD, Cotter JD, Goulet ED, Laursen PB. VIEW: is drinking to thirst adequate to appropriately maintain hydration status during prolonged endurance exercise? Yes. *Wilderness Environ Med* 2016 Jun;27(2):192–5.

86 Hoffman MD, Cotter JD, Goulet ED, Laursen PB. REBUTTAL from "Yes". *Wilderness Environ Med* 2016 Jun;27(2):198–200.

87 Armstrong LE, Johnson EC, Bergeron MF. COUNTERVIEW: is drinking to thirst adequate to appropriately maintain hydration status during prolonged endurance exercise? No. *Wilderness Environ Med* 2016 Jun;27(2):195–8.

88 Armstrong LE, Johnson EC, Bergeron MF. REBUTTAL from "No". *Wilderness Environ Med* 2016 Jun;27(2):200–2.

89 Davis JM, Burgess WA, Slentz CA, Bartoli WP, Pate RR. Effects of ingesting 6% and 12% glucose/electrolyte beverages during prolonged intermittent cycling in the heat. *Eur J Appl Physiol Occup Physiol* 1988;57(5):563–9.

90 Coyle EF. Fluid and fuel intake during exercise. *J Sports Sci* 2004 Jan;22(1):39–55.

9

HEAT-RELATED INJURY AND ILLNESS

What should you know by the end of the chapter?

Apart from compromising exercise and cognitive performance (see Chapters 4 and 5 for more details), high levels of thermal strain can pose a threat to an athlete's safety. The extent of the risk is dependent on the magnitude of thermal strain experienced which also dictates the treatment required. This chapter covers the range of thermal illness and injuries that athletes may experience and provides guidance on how to prevent and treat them. By the end of the chapter, you should know:

- What are considered heat illnesses and injuries?
- What causes the main heat illnesses and injuries?
- How can you prevent the heat injuries and illnesses occurring?
- How can you treat the different forms of heat illness and injury if they occur?

Key terms for this chapter

Core body temperature cooling rate	The rate at which core body temperatures are reduced. A cooling intervention should reduce core body temperature at a rate of at least $0.078°C\cdot min^{-1}$ (an "acceptable" cooling rate) and ideally at one in excess of $0.155°C\cdot min^{-1}$ (an "ideal" cooling rate) (1).
Endotoxemia	The presence of endotoxins in the blood caused predominantly by ischemia of the gut. The ischemia occurs as a result of blood being directed away from the gut to the skin during bouts of exercise in the

heat and increases the permeability of the paracellular cells. The increased permeability allows for the
movement of endotoxins into the circulation.

Exertional heat exhaustion	An inability to continue exercising in hot conditions usually as a result of large fluid-electrolyte losses and cardiovascular insufficiency. Athletes suffering from exertional heat exhaustion usually have rectal temperature below 40°C.
Exercise-associated muscle cramps	Often classified as a heat injury and sometimes called "exertional heat cramps" although they are not directly related to hyperthermia. Exertional heat cramps affect athletes and active workers of all ages and are painful involuntary spasms that usually only last a few seconds or minutes.
Exertional heatstroke	The most severe heat illness associated with multiple organ failure and disturbances to the central nervous system that can be fatal. Exertional heatstroke is often defined by having a core body temperature in excess of 40.5°C; however, cases have been reported when the athlete has a core body temperature lower than this. Hyperthermia appears to trigger exertional heatstroke but heatstroke is driven by an endotoxic response (see endotoxemia).
Lipopolysaccharide (LPS)	The major component of the outer membrane of gram-negative bacteria which, when released in to the circulation, can result in endotoxemia (see endotoxemia).
Sunburn	Skin damage caused by UVA and UVB rays that often results in the skin becoming warm, red, and tender.
Ultraviolet radiation	The cause of skin damage which can lead to sunburn. There are two types (UVA and UVB) which are classified based upon their wavelength.

Problem 9.1: What is wrong with your athlete?

You are the head coach of an American football team. During a very hot and strenuous preseason training camp you are informed that one of your athletes has the following symptoms – what is likely to be the problem and what should you do about it?

1   *Sweat-soaked, pale skin*
2   *Confusion*
3   *Dizziness*
4   *Headaches*
5   *Vomiting*

Problem 9.2: How can you minimise the likelihood of your athletes suffering from heat illnesses during an upcoming warm-weather training camp?

You are the head coach of an athletics club preparing to go abroad for seven days of warm-weather training. The weather at home is cold and wet, whereas it is forecast to be warm (25–32°C) and dry where you are going. What steps can you take to ensure that you minimise the risk of any of your athletes suffering from a heat illness or injury while at the training camp? The main objective of the warm-weather training camp is to escape the poor weather back home rather than to induce any heat adaptations.

9.1 Heat-related injuries

Quick question: What would you consider a heat illness or a heat injury? Have you ever experienced one? If so, what symptoms did you have? Did you require any treatment?

In addition to impairing exercise and cognitive performance (see Chapters 4 and 5), exercise-induced hyperthermia can result in the potentially dangerous heat illnesses and injuries if treatment is not rapidly administered (2;3). Heat illnesses are relatively common (4) and can range in severity from low-severity sunburn and muscle cramps to the potentially fatal exertional heatstroke. Comprehensive data relating to the incidences of heat illnesses are difficult to find because it is likely that many cases go unreported but in a recent survey, nearly half (~48%) of athletes who completed a questionnaire prior to the 2015 IAAF World Championships in Beijing reported having previously experienced at least one heat illness symptom and nearly a fifth (~17%) reported experiencing two or more (4).

Heat illness and injuries occur due to increases in tissue temperature. Externally, this might result in sunburn, but internally, an increase in tissue temperature can lead to a progressive chain of reactions, starting with minor disruptions in cellular function and potentially ending in cell death and organ failure (5;6). An internal (core body) temperature of ~40°C is often linked to the development of heat illnesses and injuries but in sufficiently motivated individuals, it is not unusual for core temperatures in excess of 40°C to be recorded following prolonged exercise in hot conditions without medical complications (7). The severity of the heat-related illness appears to be dependent upon the time spent hyperthermic rather than the peak core body temperature reached (8).

The main heat illnesses in order of increasing severity are exercise-associated muscle cramps, exertional heat exhaustion, and exertional heatstroke but this chapter will also discuss two other heat-related issues that have the potential to compromise athlete safety and exercise performance – sunburn and endotoxemia (hyponatremia which sometimes occurs during exercise in a hot environment is discussed in Chapter 8).

This section will help you to answer Problem 9.1: What is wrong with your athlete?

You are the head coach of an American football team. During a very hot and strenuous preseason training camp you are informed that one of your athletes has the following symptoms – what is likely to be the problem and what should you do about it?

1　Sweat-soaked, pale skin
2　Confusion
3　Dizziness
4　Headaches
5　Vomiting

9.1.1 Sunburn

Sunburn is not always considered a heat-illness or heat injury, but if you have ever experienced it, you will know how it can limit athletic performance. Sunburn is skin damage caused by two types of ultraviolet (UV) rays (UVA and UVB). UVB rays have a short wavelength (290–320 nm) and are the main cause of sunburn because the shorter wavelength means that UVB rays do not penetrate as deeply as UVA rays. UVA rays have a longer wavelength (320–400 nm) and are less intense that UVB despite being 30–50 times more prevalent. UVA rays penetrate the skin to a greater depth than UVB and are a major cause of skin ageing and a contributing factor to developing skin cancer. Sunburn often results in the skin initially becoming warm, red, and tender, and it may peel or flake a few days later. Although sunburn can have negative long-term effects on an athlete's health (e.g. sunburn is one of the risk factors for melanoma (9)), the immediate symptoms usually disappear within a week. Depending on the extent of the sunburn and the severity of the pain caused, sunburn may or may not have a meaningful impact on exercise performance.

Sunburn requires prolonged sun (and UV ray) exposure and so such prolonged exposure should be minimised – care should be taken not to underestimate the strength of the sun, especially if there is a strong airflow that can mask the thermal stress experienced. The environmental conditions should be considered when scheduling training and competitions as the risk of developing sunburn will differ from place to place and from time to time for example, the risk of getting sunburn is highest in the United Kingdom from March to October between 11am and 3pm.

The main risk factor for getting sunburn is being exposed to ultraviolet rays but some individuals are more susceptible than others. Holman et al. (10) recently conducted a cross-sectional study using a nationally representative sample of over 30,000 US adults examining the prevalence sunburn. Approximately one-third of responders (34.2%) reported that they had experienced sunburn in the year. Individuals of all ages and demographic background reported suffering from at least one bout of sunburn; however, the prevalence was greatest in younger (51% of adults aged 18–29 years reported having suffered from at least one bout of sunburn), non-Hispanic white individuals (43%) (10). Interestingly, Americans who engage in aerobic activity are more likely to experience sunburn than those who do not (38% versus 33%) (10) but this is probably as a result of greater sun exposure rather than any mechanistic link between increased aerobic fitness and an increased likelihood of sunburn.

9.1.2 Exercise-associated muscle cramps

Exercise-associated muscle cramps are also sometimes called "exertional heat cramps" and so are often classified as heat injuries despite the fact that they are not directly related to hyperthermia (11–13). Exertional heat cramps affect athletes and active workers of all ages and are seemingly unpredictable although some athletes report experiencing minor muscle twitches before painful cramps occur. Exertional heat cramps are relatively common (12 cases per 10,000 in marathon runners (14)) and they often result in the athlete having to stop exercising and can result in localised muscle soreness which can last for a few days post-cramp (15). As with cramps in temperate climates, the cause of exertional heat cramps is not fully understood. It has been proposed that there may be a greater incidence of heat cramps in hypohydrated athletes with low sodium concentrations (16;17); however, sweat losses, volumes ingested, and post-exercise body masses are often comparable between athletes who cramped and those that did not (12). As with other muscle cramps, the main symptoms of exertional heat cramps are painful involuntary contractions. The involuntary contractions, or spasms, usually only last a few seconds or minutes but spasms may occur for a number of hours.

9.1.3 Exertional heat exhaustion

Exertional heat exhaustion is characterised by an inability to continue exercising in hot conditions due to large fluid-electrolyte losses and cardiovascular insufficiency (5;12). The cardiovascular insufficiency appears to arise as a result of elevated cardiac output, increased peripheral vasodilation, and lowered peripheral vascular resistance leading to increased skin blood flow and subsequently low blood pressure (hypotension) (18). The frequency of exertional heat stress in athletes is unclear but it has been reported that even in mild conditions (wet-bulb globe temperature (WBGT) = 11–20°C) there are ~14 cases per 10,000 runners undertaking a 14 km road race (19). The frequency is likely to increase as heat stress increases and in addition to exercising in thermally stressful conditions (e.g. high temperature and humidity, low air flow), there are a number of risk factors that can increase the likelihood of developing exertional heat exhaustion. These include a body mass index in excess of 27 kg·m^2, and inadequate fluid consumption resulting in a state of hypohydration (20–22).

The symptoms of exertional heat exhaustion are varied and non-specific but as a result of the hypotension, athletes suffering with exertional heat exhaustion often display dizziness, fainting (heat syncope), weakness, and impaired coordination, they may feel nauseous, experience "chills", suffer muscle cramps, and often have elevated heart and breathing rates. The symptoms are similar to those associated with the more dangerous exertional heatstroke and so rectal temperature measurements should be used to distinguish between likely exertional heat exhaustion (rectal temperature <40°C) and likely exertional heatstroke (rectal temperature >40°C). If rectal temperature measurement is not possible, the condition should be considered exertional heatstroke and the appropriate treatment should be promptly initiated.

9.1.4 Exertional heatstroke

Exertional heatstroke is the most severe heat illness. Exertional heatstroke is one of the most common causes of sudden death in athletes (23); however, fortunately the incidence rates are low. It has been reported that during the first four days of American football preseason training (when athletes are especially susceptible due to lower than normal levels of fitness, intense exercise, and hot environmental conditions), there is about one case per 350,000 athletes (24) whereas the incidence rate during prolonged competitive running in warm (WBGT = 21–27°C) conditions is reported to be 10–20 cases per 10,000 runners (25).

Exertional heatstroke is often defined by severe hyperthermia (core body temperature in excess of 40.5°C), is associated with multiple organ failure and disturbances to the central nervous system (5;12), and may be triggered by systematic inflammation occurring in response to endotoxemia (see Section 9.1.5) (26). Interestingly, heatstroke can be observed at core body temperatures below 40°C and, as mentioned previously, some athletes are able to tolerate core body temperatures in excess of 40°C without obvious clinical concern (27;28). The symptoms of exertional heatstroke are wide ranging, often non-specific, and largely dependent on the extent of hyperthermia but most athletes suffering from exertional heatstroke have sweat-soaked, pale skin (5) whereas suffers of non-exertional heatstroke (sometimes referred to as classic heatstroke) often have dry, hot, and flushed skin. Other symptoms include confusion, dizziness and unusual behaviour, loss of balance, headaches, vomiting, diarrhoea, seizures, and delirium. The symptoms are very similar to those associated with exertional heat exhaustion and so in order to effectively diagnose exertional heatstroke, rectal temperature should be measured. Rectal temperature has some barriers to use but due to issues with other methods that claim to measure core body temperature (see Chapter 3 for a detailed section focusing on the pros and cons of the various measurement sites and devices), it is currently considered the best diagnostic approach.

There are a number of risk factors for exertional heatstroke and these include low aerobic fitness, poor nutritional status, a lack of heat acclimation, sunburn, sleep deprivation, age >40 years, and demanding exercise performed in highly thermally stressful conditions. Interestingly, despite poor aerobic fitness being linked to exertional heatstroke, well-trained, elite athletes can still develop the heat illness if the heat dissipation rates are insufficient to remove the heat produced by the exercise. Exertional heatstroke can occur in cool conditions (8–18°C); however, the greatest risk is posed by high-intensity exercise (>75% maximal oxygen uptake) performed in WBGTs exceeding 28°C (5). Unsurprisingly, poor health status increases the risk of developing exertional heatstroke and so athletes should not exercise in the heat if they are suffering from a fever or a respiratory infection, have diarrhoea, or are vomiting.

9.1.5 Endotoxemia

Endotoxemia describes the presence of endotoxins (more specifically lipopolysaccharides (LPS)) in the blood rather than where they are usually found – in the gram-negative bacteria located in the small and large intestines. Endotoxemia can be triggered by exercise alone but it is exacerbated by hyperthermia and is thought to be a major cause of heatstroke (26). The main reason that hyperthermia and exercise seem to induce an endotoxic state is due to the redistribution of blood flow. The gut region is one area that suffers greatly from the redistribution of blood flow during hyperthermia as blood is redirected from the core to the periphery to facilitate heat loss. Gut blood flow is reduced by ~80% during exercise (29) and this reduction is even greater during hyperthermia (30). The reduced blood flow to the gut results in localised ischemia and the breakdown of the gut cell membrane. The breakdown of the gut cell membrane increases the permeability of the paracellular cells allowing previously contained LPS fragments from intestinal gram-negative bacteria (which are harmless if contained) to move into the circulation. The movement of the endotoxins from the gut into the circulation causes a systemic inflammatory response that increases the risk of endotoxemic shock. The endotoxemia model of heat stoke suggests that while hyperthermia is the trigger, the heatstroke is driven by the systemic inflammation and septicaemia (26) that occurs due to endotoxemia.

Quick question: At the start of this section I asked whether you had ever experienced a heat illness or injury – did you answer "no"? Many go undiagnosed, so do you think you would change your answer now?

9.2 Preventing heat illness and injuries

This section will help you to address Problem 9.2: How can you minimise the likelihood of your athletes suffering from heat illnesses during an upcoming warm-weather training camp?

You are the head coach of an athletics club preparing to go abroad for seven days of warm-weather training. The weather at home is cold and wet whereas it is forecast to be warm (25–32°C) and dry where you are going. What steps can you take to ensure that you minimise the risk of any of your athletes suffering from a heat illness or injury while at the training camp? The main objective of the warm-weather training camp is to escape the poor weather back home rather than to induce any heat adaptations.

As a result of the potentially fatal consequences of exertional heat illnesses, the best course of action is to prevent its onset (12). Effective prevention strategies include cancelling, postponing, or rescheduling sporting events in particularly dangerous environmental conditions to avoid the sun (see Chapter 3), applying sunscreen, wearing clothing that covers the skin, pre-exercise screening to identify at risk individuals, and undertaking an effective heat acclimation regimen prior to subsequent heat exposure (see Chapter 6). Hypohydration and low sodium concentrations may be a trigger for exertional muscle cramps (16;17) (although this is an area of debate) and so maintaining a euhydrated state may offer some protection. Sunburn can easily be avoided and the most commonly used ways to do so are staying in the shade (~37% of responders), wearing sunscreen (~32% of responders), and wearing long clothing to cover the skin (~28% of responders) (10). Unsurprisingly, simply avoiding the sun (e.g. by rescheduling activities for the cooler parts of the day or seeking shade) and applying sunscreen both reduce the incidence of sunburn (10). When using sunscreen, the National Health Service of the United Kingdom recommends that sunscreen should be water resistant (to avoid sweat-loss washing it off), it should provide at least four-star UVA protection, and it should have a sun protection factor (commonly abbreviated to SPF on sun cream) of at least 15 to protect against UVB radiation.

Hyperthermia is a key trigger for exertional heat illnesses and injuries so the best way to prevent their development is to take steps to prevent hyperthermia occurring. Avoiding heat illness need not be too disruptive and can be achieved with relatively minor changes. For example, American Football players appear especially susceptible to exertional heatstroke during the first four days of pre-season training which often take place in the most thermally stressful period of the year and at a time that the players are attempting to regain fitness. American football players have the added risk factor of highly insulative clothing and so coaches should consider reducing the intensity of the training, rescheduling the time of training for the cooler mornings and/or evenings, and reducing the clothing worn during such practices (e.g. conduct as much non-contact practice as possible without the pads and helmets) (Figure 9.1).

In addition to hyperthermia, exertional heat illnesses are related to the inflammatory response and septicaemia that occurs as a result of the endotoxic response to exercise and hyperthermia. This response can be prevented to some degree by maintaining a "normal" core body temperature; however, limiting core body temperature increases may not be desirable (e.g. if you are trying to acclimate your athletes to the heat stress) and even if it is desirable, severe heat illnesses can occur at core body temperatures below 40°C. Several nutritional strategies have been proposed to help maintain gut integrity (and therefore reduce the LPS release). The strategies that appear effective include vitamin C (31), probiotics (32), glutamine (33), carbohydrates (34), and protein (34) (although the effect of protein appears minimal (34)) and so supplementation with these may offer some protection against endotoxemia. Conversely, antiinflammatory medications (e.g. ibuprofen) appear to aggravate exercise-induced

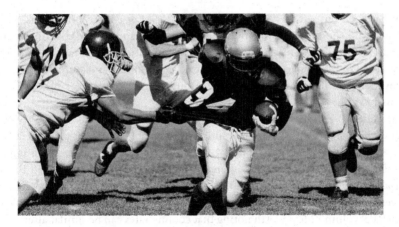

FIGURE 9.1 American football player in full kit.

gastrointestinal injury (35) and so should be avoided as they may increase the risk of endotoxemia if consumed during or prior to exercise in the heat.

9.3 Treating heat illnesses and injuries

If heat illnesses do occur (despite adopting prevention strategies or because such strategies were not adopted), the required treatment is dependent upon the severity of the heat illness.

9.3.1 Treating minor heat illnesses and injuries

The symptoms of sunburn cannot really be treated but the pain associated with them can be managed. Cooling the skin (e.g. by having a cold shower or applying a cold flannel to the site) and moisturising the skin with lotions containing aloe vera is a good idea. Exertional heat cramps and exhaustion can be treated with rest, stretching, and sodium chloride ingestion (in food and/or beverages) (5) but in some severe cases intravenous saline infusion (saline is a mixture of sodium chloride and water often used in clinical settings) may be required. Exertional heat cramps may also occur as a result of hyponatremia (see Chapter 8 for more information on hyponatremia) and so measurements of plasma or serum sodium concentrations should be performed to confirm the appropriate diagnosis before large volumes of fluid are administered.

9.3.2 Treating major heat illnesses and injuries

Although minor heat illnesses can usually be treated with supine rest in the shade (additional skin cooling and/or rehydration can be administered if required), more severe heat illnesses require the rapid reduction of body temperature to <38.9°C (12). This reduction should ideally occur within 30 min (36) – a period that has been termed the "golden half hour" (11). For effective diagnosis, rectal temperature should be recorded as soon as possible and it should be monitored throughout recovery. In addition to rectal temperature, heart rate, blood pressure, and cognitive performance should be continuously measured during the recovery phase to give information regarding the restoration (or otherwise) of normal cardiovascular and cognitive function.

In order to rapidly reduce core body temperature from >40.5°C to <38.9°C (12) within ~30 min (36), an intervention must be able to cool at a rate of at least $0.05°C \cdot min^{-1}$ (a reduction of at least 1.6°C in 30 min). The term *at least* is important here because time is of the essence. McDermott et al. (1) suggested that an *acceptable* cooling rate is actually $0.078–0.155°C \cdot min^{-1}$ whereas an *ideal* cooling intervention would cool at a rate of at least $0.155°C \cdot min^{-1}$ – both faster cooling rates than $0.05°C \cdot min^{-1}$. It is worth noting that cooling rates can be similar after delays of 5 ($0.20°C \cdot min^{-1}$), 20 ($0.17°C \cdot min^{-1}$), and 40 ($0.17°C \cdot min^{-1}$) min (37) and so although cooling should ideally be administered, immediately cooling should still be administered as soon as possible if immediate treatment cannot be provided.

A wide range of post-exercise cooling interventions (e.g. ice sheets, ice towels, cold showers, forearm immersion, and cooling garments) are used to cool hyperthermic athletes but the cooling rate provided by these practical interventions often falls well below the acceptable and ideal cooling rates. Examples of some of the reported cooling rates are as follows (Table 9.1):

Forearm cooling is often purported to be effective (and is regularly used in occupational settings such as firefighting) but the overall cooling rate is slow (0.01 and $0.04°C \cdot min^{-1}$ (38–42)). Initial cooling rates can be faster (e.g. Maroni et al. (43) observed cooling rates of ~$0.07–0.10°C \cdot min^{-1}$ in the first 15 min of a 30 min cooling bout) but the cooling rate slows rapidly (~$0.04°C\ min^{-1}$ after 30 min). As with pre-cooling (see Chapter 7), the most effective way to cool an athlete post-exercise is by immersing the whole body in water. In a comprehensive review, Zhang et al. (44) reported that the mean cooling rate of water immersion was $0.08 \pm 0.03°C \cdot min^{-1}$. This cooling rate is twice as fast as the mean cooling

TABLE 9.1 Summary of practical cooling interventions and their effectiveness

Cooling method	Reported cooling rate(s)	Cooling rate classification using the McDermott et al. (1) classifications
Forearm or hand cold-water immersion	$0.01–0.04°C \cdot min^{-1}$ (38–42)	Unacceptable
Passive rest	$0.01–0.05°C \cdot min^{-1}$ (43–45)	Unacceptable
Cold packs	$0.02–0.06°C \cdot min^{-1}$ (44)	Unacceptable
Ice vests	$0.03–0.05°C \cdot min^{-1}$ (46;47)	Unacceptable
Ice sheet cooling	$0.05°C \cdot min^{-1}$ (43)	Unacceptable
Ice towel application	$0.06–0.11°C \cdot min^{-1}$ (48;49)	Possibly acceptable
Cold showers	$0.07°C \cdot min^{-1}$ (43)	Unacceptable

rate of passive recovery alone ($0.04°C·min^{-1}$) and of the most effective forearm/ hand cold-water immersion trials, and falls in the *acceptable* but not *ideal* classifications of McDermott et al. (1).

On average, cold-water immersion is most effective at lowering core body temperature when body temperatures are higher ($\geq38.6°C$), water temperatures are lower ($\leq10°C$), ambient temperatures are $\geq20°C$, immersion durations are ≤10 min, and when the torso and limbs are both immersed (44). Using the mean data reported by Zhang et al. (44), the mean time taken to cool the body by $1°C$ in otherwise healthy, moderately hyperthermic individuals can be as little as 5 min or as long as 22 min depending on the starting core body temperature, the temperature of the water used, and the extent of the immersion (Figure 9.2 (44)), with the most effective cooling occurring when very hyperthermic (core body temperature $>40°C$) individuals are fully immersed in cold ($<5°C$) water.

Although the data from Zhang et al. (44) suggest otherwise, as mentioned in Chapter 7, when it comes to the water temperature to use for water immersion it is not always a case of "the colder the better" because if the water is too cold, peripheral vasoconstriction can reduce peripheral blood flow and limit the transfer of heat between the water and the skin. Very cold water is also often poorly tolerated by athletes. Immersing an athlete in very cold water (~2°C) can result in very fast cooling rates (45–47); however, warmer water may be comparatively effective (48). Cooling rates using water at 9.2°C ($0.17°C·min^{-1}$ (49)) are faster than using water at 2.0°C ($0.14°C·min^{-1}$ (50)) and interestingly oesophageal temperature can be rapidly reduced using even warmer water (26°C) (48). In this study, hyperthermic participants (they had a

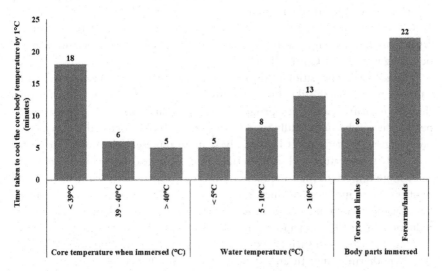

FIGURE 9.2 Mean time taken to cool the core body temperature by 1°C. Redrawn from data contained in Zhang et al. (44).

core body temperature of 39.5°C) were cooled at a rate of 0.10°C·min^{-1} in cool air (~23°C), 0.88°C·min^{-1} in cold (14°C) water, and 0.71°C min^{-1} when using cool (26°C) water (48). The authors converted these cooling rates into the estimated time required to lower the hyperthermic core body temperature (39.5°C) to 37.5°C and noted that although the 14°C water was quicker (2.2 ± 0.7 min), the difference between 14°C water and 26°C water (2.9 ± 1.2 min) was minimal (~0.7 min or ~42 s). Unsurprisingly, both water immersion trials were ~20 min quicker than the passive control although the rate observed by passive rest was highly variable (22.8 ± 16.4 min) (48). Small differences between the cooling rates of cold and cool water have been reported elsewhere by the same research group (51), but the rates reported in these two studies are much faster than reported elsewhere. For example, it was reported elsewhere that water at 20°C took on average ~17 min to cool a hyperthermic individual (46) – much longer than the ~2.5 min reported. As discussed at length in Chapter 3, core body temperature is far from homogenous and the temperatures recorded will differ between sites and as a result of different measurement approaches being taken. In the case of the post-exercise cooling rates reported here, the large difference appears to be due to the different sites of measurement. Rectal temperature is most commonly used but when Proulx et al. (52) compared the rate of cooling measured at the oesophagus with that measured rectally, they found that the rate of cooling was greater when measured at the oesophagus (Figure 9.3). The slower times required to reduce core body temperature to ~37.5°C (~17 min) was reported when rectal temperature was used as a measurement of core body temperature (46), whereas the shorter periods of time (~3 min) were observed when oesophageal temperature was used (48;51). Rectal temperature cooling rates depend upon water temperature, with the faster rates being observed when colder temperatures are used (2°C = 0.35°C min^{-1}; 8°C = 0.19°C min^{-1}; 14°C = 0.15°C min^{-1}; 20°C = 0.19°C min^{-1}), whereas cooling rates are similar regardless of water temperature when core body temperature is measured at the oesophagus (0.6–1.0°C min^{-1}) (52).

There is often opposition to the measurement of rectal temperature from athletes and practitioners alike due to the invasive nature (53) but it is less invasive than the measurement of oesophageal temperature and unlike oesophageal temperature it can be successfully used in the field (54). As discussed in Chapter 3, oesophageal temperature is likely to be a more representative temperature for core body temperature and so reductions in oesophageal temperature are likely to be more important than a reduction in rectal temperature. While using rectal temperature to monitor an athlete's recovery from a hyperthermic state, remember that the reduction in oesophageal temperature is very likely to exceed this reduction in rectal temperature, and awareness of this is required to prevent cooling the athletes to such an extent that they move from a hyperthermic state to a hypothermic one. In an experiment that simultaneously measured rectal and oesophageal temperature, Proulx et al. (52) reported that by the time rectal temperature had been reduced to 37.7°C, oesophageal temperature was actually 33.9°C. The authors recommended that when using very cold (2–8°C) or cold

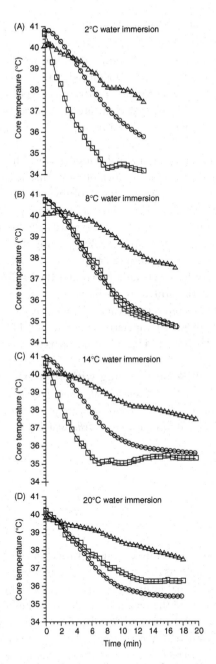

FIGURE 9.3 Representative core body temperatures during immersion at water temperatures of 2°C (a), 8°C (b), 14°C (c), and 20°C (d) for one participant (52). Open box = oesophageal temperature; open circle = aural canal temperature; and open triangle = rectal temperature. Reprinted by permission from Springer Nature: European Journal of Applied Physiology. Proulx et al. (52). Safe cooling limits from exercise-induced hyperthermia. *Eur J Appl Physiol* 2006 Mar;96(4):434–45. Springer 2006.

(14–20°C) water to cool hyperthermic athletes, the target rectal temperatures should be adjusted to 38.6°C and 37.8°C, respectively, to effectively reduce core body temperature without causing hypothermia. It is worth noting that because severe heat illnesses are often observed alongside other physiological issues (e.g. circulatory failure), the rate at which an extremely hyperthermic athlete cools can be as little as ~20% of the expected rate (3) and so the rates observed in the field may be lower than those cited here which are from the experimental literature.

Post-exercise water immersion can be logistically difficult (and sometimes even impossible) but there are a number of ways that it can be administered. Rigid structures, such as specialist cooling pools, wheelie bins, and bathtubs, can also be used, and tarp cooling offers a potentially more practical method (especially for clubs with limited resources) because tarps are often less expensive and easier to store and move. Tarp cooling involves placing the hyperthermic athlete on a waterproof sheet (i.e. a tarpaulin or "tarp"), having at least three individuals hold up the edges in order to create a bowl, and then filling the "bowl" with cold/iced water. Once the athlete is in the water, if the water is agitated (i.e. moved about to facilitate convective heat exchange), this form of cold-water immersion can reduce core body temperature at a rate of 0.14°C min^{-1} and 0.17°C min^{-1} with water at 2°C (50) and 9.2°C (49), respectively.

Problem 9.1 revisited: What is wrong with your athlete?

You are the head coach of an American football team. During a very hot and strenuous preseason training camp you are informed that one of your athletes has the following symptoms – what is likely to be the problem and what should you do about it?

1   *Sweat-soaked, pale skin*
2   *Confusion*
3   *Dizziness*
4   *Headaches*
5   *Vomiting*

Although the symptoms of heat illness can be varied and non-specific, the severity of these symptoms suggests that your athlete is either suffering from exertional heat exhaustion or exertional heatstroke. The symptoms of the two more severe heat illnesses are similar and the recommended way to differentiate between the two is to measure the rectal core body temperature of the athlete. If you have a trained physician on your staff, rectal temperature should be swiftly measured as this will allow for the correct diagnosis – if rectal temperature is below 40°C, exertional heat exhaustion is the most likely diagnosis but if rectal temperature is higher than this the athlete is likely to be suffering from exertional heatstroke (although debate exists regarding the importance of core body temperature in the onset of exertional heatstroke (26), its measurement is still considered the best practice currently). Exertional heatstroke is associated with multiple organ failure and disturbances to the central nervous system (5;12) and so treatment needs to be swift and effective. If rectal temperature measurement is not possible, the condition should be considered exertional heatstroke and the appropriate treatment should be promptly initiated.

If core body temperature is below 40°C and a diagnosis of exertional heat exhaustion is made, the cessation of exercise and supine rest in the shade is likely to be sufficient. Additional skin cooling and/or rehydration can be administered if required.

If core body temperature exceeds 40°C (or if rectal temperature assessment is unavailable and the symptoms are being treated as exertional heatstroke), core body temperature should ideally be reduced to below 38.9°C (12) within 30 min (36). The emergency services should be called and cooling should be immediately initiated. Whole-body water immersion is the most effective cooling method and so should be adopted if possible – if a specialist immersion facility or item (e.g. cooling pool, bathtub, wheelie bin) is not available, tarp cooling can be used. The water needs to be colder than the athlete in order to facilitate heat transfer but it need not be very cold and so cold tap water is likely to be sufficient if you are able to monitor rectal temperature; during the recovery phase, you can manipulate the temperature of the water based on the cooling rate observed i.e. if it is too slow you should aim to cool the water perhaps by adding ice. Remember that rectal temperature cools at a slower rate than oesophageal temperature and so to prevent hypothermia the target rectal temperatures should be 38.6°C and 37.8°C, respectively, when using very cold (2–8°C) or cold (14–20°C) water (52).

Cooling approaches that do not use water immersion are far less effective but if whole-body water immersion is impossible, other cooling approaches such as localised limb immersion, cold towel application, and water dousing can be used to offer some cooling prior to the arrival of the emergency services. Heart rate, blood pressure, and cognitive performance should be continuously measured during the recovery phase regardless or not of whether rectal temperature is being monitored.

Problem 9.2 revisited: How can you minimise the likelihood of your athletes suffering from heat illnesses during an upcoming warm-weather training camp?

You are the head coach of an athletics club preparing to go abroad for seven days of warm-weather training. The weather at home is cold and wet whereas it is forecast to be warm (25–32°C) and dry where you are going. What steps can you take to ensure that you minimise the risk of any of your athletes suffering from a heat illness or injury while at the training camp? The main objective of the warm-weather training camp is to escape the poor weather back home rather than to induce any heat adaptations.

An important thing to consider here is that the goal of the warm-weather training camp is not to induce beneficial adaptations to heat (i.e. heat acclimatisation) and so you can take a cautious approach when it comes to heat exposure. If you were aiming to acclimatise your athletes to heat their health should still be a priority but you would need to balance the risk of developing a heat illness with the need to provide a sufficient thermal impulse (i.e. increase in core body temperature) to see physiological adaptation (see Chapter 6 for more information on heat acclimation and acclimatisation).

There are a number of potentially effective strategies that you can adopt to minimise the risk of any of your athletes developing a heat illness and these should all be considered:

- You should screen your athletes prior to leaving to establish whether any of them may be especially susceptible. Any athletes who report any of the following should be closely monitored:
  - Low aerobic fitness
  - Poor nutritional status
  - A lack of heat acclimation
  - Sunburn
  - Sleep deprivation
  - Age >40 years
  - A fever
  - A respiratory infection
  - Diarrhoea
  - Vomiting
- If possible, undertaking a progressive heat acclimation regimen prior to flying out would be a good idea (see Chapter 6 for more information on heat acclimation regimens).
- Training should be planned so that it avoids the sun as much as possible. This can easily be achieved scheduling activities for the cooler parts of the day or undertaking them indoors or in shaded areas.
- When exposed to the sun, your athletes should apply sufficient water-resistant sunscreen to all exposed skin. The sunscreen should provide at least four-star UVA protection and have a sun protection factor (commonly abbreviated to SPF on sunscreen) of at least 15.
- Make sure that your athletes wear clothing that facilitates heat loss. Any heat-restrictive items (e.g. helmets, overalls, or pads) should be removed where possible or used only when the heat stress levels are low.
- Ensure that your athletes maintain a euhydrated state and consume foods or fluids that also contain sodium may offer some protection against heat cramps (see Chapter 8 for more on athlete hydration).
- Your athletes should consume a diet containing vitamin C, probiotics, glutamine, and carbohydrates.
- Athletes should avoid taking anti-inflammatory medications (e.g. ibuprofen) unless absolutely necessary.

9.4 Summary

Exercising in hot conditions can pose a threat to an athlete's health, especially if the athlete is out of shape (low levels of aerobic fitness), ageing (over 40), already ill, and/or non-heat acclimated. The most effective ways to prevent heat illnesses of injuries occurring is to ensure that the athlete is covered up as much as possible (with lightweight clothing), is wearing sunscreen, and avoids the sun as much as possible (e.g. training can be rescheduled for cooler mornings or evenings rather than in the afternoon). Heat illness and injuries range in severity from the relatively minor sunburn (although sunburn can increase the likelihood of developing skin cancer later in life and so should not be considered "minor") to the potentially fatal exertional heatstroke. Swift diagnosis and treatment are required to minimise the complications associated with heat illness or injuries and minor heat illnesses are often treated with shaded rest and rehydration whereas more severe heat illnesses such as exertional heatstroke require the rapid reduction of core body temperature. There are many ways to cool the body; however, only whole-body water immersion cools at a sufficiently fast rate. If whole-body water immersion is not possible, other methods (e.g. cold towel application, partial water immersion) can be used while the emergency services are on their way but if there is a high risk of heat illnesses occurring, water-immersion facilities should be provided – this need not involve specialist immersion tubs as tarps can effectively be used.

9.5 Self-check quiz

At the beginning of this chapter you were told that by this point you should know the answers to the following broad questions:

- What are considered heat illnesses and injuries?
- What causes the main heat illnesses and injuries?
- How can you prevent the heat injuries and illnesses occurring?
- How can you treat the different forms of heat illness and injury if they occur?

In order to see whether you do now know the answers to these questions, have a go at this short self-check quiz. The answers follow the questions, but before looking at the answers, if you are stuck on any question, try looking back at the relevant section. For help with questions 1–5, take another look at Section 9.1; if you are stuck on question 6, take another look at Section 9.2; and if questions 7–10 are causing you a headache, the answers can be found in Section 9.3.

9.5.1 Self-check quiz questions

1. Which type of ultraviolet radiation is the main cause of sunburn?
2. What are exertional heat cramps also known as?

3. What is exertional heat exhaustion?
4. What is the most likely heat illness if your athlete is dizzy, light-headed, vomiting, and has a rectal temperature of 40.9°C?
5. What causes endotoxemia during exercise in the heat?
6. Name three ways to prevent the onset of heat illnesses.
7. What is the best way to treat sunburn?
8. What is the best way to treat exertional heat exhaustion or exertional heat cramps?
9. What is an acceptable cooling rate for core body temperature?
10. What temperature cools more rapidly during whole-body cold-water immersion – rectal or oesophageal?

9.5.2 Self-check quiz answers

1. UVB.
2. Exercise-associated muscle cramps.
3. Exertional heat exhaustion is often defined as an inability to continue exercising in hot conditions due to large fluid-electrolyte losses and cardiovascular insufficiency.
4. Exertional heatstroke.
5. Reduced blood flow to the gut region leads to a state of localised hypoxia and increases the permeability of paracellular cells. The increased permeability results in the movement of lipopolysaccharide fragments from intestinal gram-negative bacteria into the circulation.
6. Prevention methods include avoiding the sun/hottest parts of the day; applying sunscreen with at least four-star UVA protection and a sun protection factor of at least 15; covering up with clothing (e.g. by wearing long-sleeved clothing and wide-brimmed hats); undertaking heat acclimation; removing insulative clothing; staying hydrated; and ensuring that your athlete's diet contains vitamin C, probiotics, glutamine, and carbohydrates.
7. Move in to shade, apply moisturiser with Aloe Vera, and avoid subsequent sun exposure.
8. Supine rest in a shaded place. Fluids containing sodium can be administered if required/desired.
9. McDermott et al. (1) suggested that an acceptable cooling rate is 0.078–0.155°C min^{-1} (an ideal cooling rate is at least 0.155°C min^{-1}).
10. Oesophageal temperature cools more rapidly and this should be considered when cooling a hyperthermic athlete to prevent overcooling.

9.6 Practical toolkit

Table 9.2 summaries the causes, symptoms, and treatment for sunburn, exertional heat cramps, heat exhaustion, and heat stroke.

TABLE 9.2 Heat illness quick reference table: causes, symptoms, and treatment

	Sunburn	Exertional heat cramps	Heat exhaustion	Heatstroke
Description	Skin damage caused by ultraviolet radiation. The skin is usually warm, red, and tender once burnt	Acute, painful, involuntary muscle spasms	Inability to continue exercise in the heat due to cardiovascular insufficiency	A potential fatal condition caused by hyperthermia and endotoxemia
Cause	• Prolonged exposure to the sun without adequate protection	• Hypohydration • Low sodium concentrations • Muscular fatigue	• Elevated core body temperature (usually <40°C)	• Severe hyperthermia (usually a core body temperature >40.5°C) • Systemic inflammation • Septicaemia
Treatment	• Pain management e.g. moisturiser with Aloe Vera and cool towels	• Cease exercise • Seek shade • Consume fluids with added sodium	• Cease exercise • Seek shade • Apply cooling if required • Consume fluids with added sodium	• Immediate cold/cool water immersion • Reduce core body temperature to <38.9°C
Recovery time frame	• A few days to about a week depending on severity	• Minutes to hours	• Usually within 24 hours • Same day return to play should be avoided	• Depends on the speed and effectiveness of treatment

References

1 McDermott BP, Casa DJ, Ganio MS, Lopez RM, Yeargin SW, Armstrong LE, et al. Acute whole-body cooling for exercise-induced hyperthermia: a systematic review. *J Athl Train* 2009 Jan;44(1):84–93.
2 Epstein Y, Roberts WO, Golan R, Heled Y, Sorkine P, Halpern P. Sepsis, septic shock, and fatal exertional heat stroke. *Curr Sports Med Rep* 2015 Jan;14(1):64–9.
3 Rae DE, Knobel GJ, Mann T, Swart J, Tucker R, Noakes TD. Heatstroke during endurance exercise: is there evidence for excessive endothermy? *Med Sci Sports Exerc* 2008 Jul;40(7):1193–204.
4 Periard JD, Racinais S, Timpka T, Dahlstrom O, Spreco A, Jacobsson J, et al. Strategies and factors associated with preparing for competing in the heat: a cohort study at the 2015 IAAF World Athletics Championships. *Br J Sports Med* 2017 Feb;51(4):264–70.

5 Armstrong LE, Casa DJ, Millard-Stafford M, Moran DS, Pyne SW, Roberts WO. American college of sports medicine position stand. Exertional heat illness during training and competition. *Med Sci Sports Exerc* 2007 Mar;39(3):556–72.

6 Lambert EV, St Clair GA, Noakes TD. Complex systems model of fatigue: integrative homoeostatic control of peripheral physiological systems during exercise in humans. *Br J Sports Med* 2005 Jan;39(1):52–62.

7 Webb P. Afterdrop of body temperature during rewarming: an alternative explanation. *J Appl Physiol* 1986 Feb;60(2):385–90.

8 Costrini A. Emergency treatment of exertional heatstroke and comparison of whole body cooling techniques. *Med Sci Sports Exerc* 1990 Feb;22(1):15–8.

9 Hoel DG, Berwick M, de Gruijl FR, Holick MF. The risks and benefits of sun exposure 2016. *Dermatoendocrinol* 2016 Jan;8(1):e1248325.

10 Holman DM, Ding H, Guy GP, Jr., Watson M, Hartman AM, Perna FM. Prevalence of sun protection use and sunburn and association of demographic and behaviorial characteristics with sunburn among US Adults. *JAMA Dermatol* 2018 May 1;154(5):561–8.

11 Casa DJ, Armstrong LE, Kenny GP, O'Connor FG, Huggins RA. Exertional heat stroke: new concepts regarding cause and care. *Curr Sports Med Rep* 2012 May;11(3):115–23.

12 Casa DJ, DeMartini JK, Bergeron MF, Csillan D, Eichner ER, Lopez RM, et al. National athletic trainers' association position statement: exertional heat illnesses. *J Athl Train* 2015 Sep;50(9):986–1000.

13 Maughan RJ. Exercise-induced muscle cramp: a prospective biochemical study in marathon runners. *J Sports Sci* 1986;4(1):31–4.

14 Roberts WO. A 12-yr profile of medical injury and illness for the twin cities marathon. *Med Sci Sports Exerc* 2000 Sep;32(9):1549–55.

15 Maquirriain J, Merello M. The athlete with muscular cramps: clinical approach. *J Am Acad Orthop Surg* 2007 Jul;15(7):425–31.

16 Bergeron MF. Heat cramps during tennis: a case report. *Int J Sport Nutr* 1996 Mar;6(1):62–8.

17 Bergeron MF. Heat cramps: fluid and electrolyte challenges during tennis in the heat. *J Sci Med Sport* 2003 Mar;6(1):19–27.

18 Shahid MS, Hatle L, Mansour H, Mimish L. Echocardiographic and Doppler study of patients with heatstroke and heat exhaustion. *Int J Card Imaging* 1999 Aug;15(4):279–85.

19 Richards R, Richards D. Exertion-induced heat exhaustion and other medical aspects of the city-to-surf fun runs, 1978–1984. *Med J Aust* 1984 Dec 8;141(12–13):799–805.

20 Donoghue AM, Bates GP. The risk of heat exhaustion at a deep underground metalliferous mine in relation to body-mass index and predicted VO2max. *Occup Med (Lond)* 2000 May;50(4):259–63.

21 Donoghue AM, Bates GP. The risk of heat exhaustion at a deep underground metalliferous mine in relation to surface temperatures. *Occup Med (Lond)* 2000 Jul;50(5):334–6.

22 Donoghue AM, Sinclair MJ, Bates GP. Heat exhaustion in a deep underground metalliferous mine. *Occup Environ Med* 2000 Mar;57(3):165–74.

23 Kerr ZY, Casa DJ, Marshall SW, Comstock RD. Epidemiology of exertional heat illness among U.S. high school athletes. *Am J Prev Med* 2013 Jan;44(1):8–14.

24 Roberts WO. Common threads in a random tapestry: another viewpoint on exertional heatstroke. *Phys Sportsmed* 2005 Oct;33(10):42–9.

25 Brodeur VB, Dennett SR, Griffin LS. Exertional hyperthermia, ice baths, and emergency care at the Falmouth road race. *J Emerg Nurs* 1989 Jul;15(4):304–12.

26 Lim CL, Mackinnon LT. The roles of exercise-induced immune system disturbances in the pathology of heat stroke: the dual pathway model of heat stroke. *Sports Med* 2006;36(1):39–64.

27 Muldoon S, Deuster P, Brandom B, Bunger R. Is there a link between malignant hyperthermia and exertional heat illness? *Exerc Sport Sci Rev* 2004 Oct;32(4):174–9.

28 Shibolet S, Lancaster MC, Danon Y. Heat stroke: a review. *Aviat Space Environ Med* 1976 Mar;47(3):280–301.

29 Clausen JP. Effect of physical training on cardiovascular adjustments to exercise in man. *Physiol Rev* 1977 Oct;57(4):779–815.

30 Sakurada S, Hales JR. A role for gastrointestinal endotoxins in enhancement of heat tolerance by physical fitness. *J Appl Physiol (1985)* 1998 Jan;84(1):207–14.

31 Ashton T, Young IS, Davison GW, Rowlands CC, McEneny J, Van BC, et al. Exercise-induced endotoxemia: the effect of ascorbic acid supplementation. *Free Radic Biol Med* 2003 Aug 1;35(3):284–91.

32 Shing CM, Peake JM, Lim CL, Briskey D, Walsh NP, Fortes MB, et al. Effects of probiotics supplementation on gastrointestinal permeability, inflammation and exercise performance in the heat. *Eur J Appl Physiol* 2014 Jan;114(1):93–103.

33 Pugh JN, Sage S, Hutson M, Doran DA, Fleming SC, Highton J, et al. Glutamine supplementation reduces markers of intestinal permeability during running in the heat in a dose-dependent manner. *Eur J Appl Physiol* 2017 Dec;117(12):2569–77.

34 Snipe RMJ, Khoo A, Kitic CM, Gibson PR, Costa RJS. Carbohydrate and protein intake during exertional heat stress ameliorates intestinal epithelial injury and small intestine permeability. *Appl Physiol Nutr Metab* 2017 Dec;42(12):1283–92.

35 van WK, Lenaerts K, Van Bijnen AA, Boonen B, van Loon LJ, Dejong CH, et al. Aggravation of exercise-induced intestinal injury by Ibuprofen in athletes. *Med Sci Sports Exerc* 2012 Dec;44(12):2257–62.

36 Adams WM, Hosokawa Y, Casa DJ. The timing of exertional heat stroke survival starts prior to collapse. *Curr Sports Med Rep* 2015 Jul;14(4):273–4.

37 Flouris AD, Friesen BJ, Carlson MJ, Casa DJ, Kenny GP. Effectiveness of cold water immersion for treating exertional heat stress when immediate response is not possible. *Scand J Med Sci Sports* 2015 Jun;25 Suppl 1:229–39.

38 Adams EL, Vandermark LW, Pryor JL, Pryor RR, VanScoy RM, Denegar CR, et al. Effects of heat acclimation on hand cooling efficacy following exercise in the heat. *J Sports Sci* 2017 May;35(9):828–34.

39 Adams WM, Hosokawa Y, Adams EL, Belval LN, Huggins RA, Casa DJ. Reduction in body temperature using hand cooling versus passive rest after exercise in the heat. *J Sci Med Sport* 2016 Nov;19(11):936–40.

40 Grahn DA, Dillon JL, Heller HC. Heat loss through the glabrous skin surfaces of heavily insulated, heat-stressed individuals. *J Biomech Eng* 2009 Jul;131(7):071005.

41 Hostler D, Reis SE, Bednez JC, Kerin S, Suyama J. Comparison of active cooling devices with passive cooling for rehabilitation of firefighters performing exercise in thermal protective clothing: a report from the Fireground Rehab Evaluation (FIRE) trial. *Prehosp Emerg Care* 2010 Jul;14(3):300–9.

42 Kuennen MR, Gillum TL, Amorim FT, Kwon YS, Schneider SM. Palm cooling to reduce heat strain in subjects during simulated armoured vehicle transport. *Eur J Appl Physiol* 2010 Apr;108(6):1217–23.

43 Maroni T, Dawson B, Barnett K, Guelfi K, Brade C, Naylor L, et al. Effectiveness of hand cooling and a cooling jacket on post-exercise cooling rates in hyperthermic athletes. *Eur J Sport Sci* 2018 Jan 24;18:1–9.

44 Zhang Y, Davis JK, Casa DJ, Bishop PA. Optimizing cold water immersion for exercise-induced hyperthermia: a meta-analysis. *Med Sci Sports Exerc* 2015 Nov;47(11):2464–72.

45 Friesen BJ, Carter MR, Poirier MP, Kenny GP. Water immersion in the treatment of exertional hyperthermia: physical determinants. *Med Sci Sports Exerc* 2014 Sep;46(9):1727–35.

46 Proulx CI, Ducharme MB, Kenny GP. Effect of water temperature on cooling efficiency during hyperthermia in humans. *J Appl Physiol (1985)* 2003 Apr;94(4):1317–23.

47 Tan PM, Teo EY, Ali NB, Ang BC, Iskandar I, Law LY, et al. Evaluation of various cooling systems after exercise-induced hyperthermia. *J Athl Train* 2017 Feb;52(2):108–16.

48 Taylor NA, Caldwell JN, Van den Heuvel AM, Patterson MJ. To cool, but not too cool: that is the question--immersion cooling for hyperthermia. *Med Sci Sports Exerc* 2008 Nov;40(11):1962–9.

49 Hosokawa Y, Adams WM, Belval LN, Vandermark LW, Casa DJ. Tarp-assisted cooling as a method of whole-body cooling in hyperthermic individuals. *Ann Emerg Med* 2017 Mar;69(3):347–52.

50 Luhring KE, Butts CL, Smith CR, Bonacci JA, Ylanan RC, Ganio MS, et al. Cooling effectiveness of a modified cold-water immersion method after exercise-induced hyperthermia. *J Athl Train* 2016 Nov;51(11):946–51.

51 Caldwell JN, van den Heuvel AMJ, Kerry P, Clark MJ, Peoples GE, Taylor NAS. A vascular mechanism to explain thermally mediated variations in deep-body cooling rates during the immersion of profoundly hyperthermic individuals. *Exp Physiol* 2018 Apr;103:512–22.

52 Proulx CI, Ducharme MB, Kenny GP. Safe cooling limits from exercise-induced hyperthermia. *Eur J Appl Physiol* 2006 Mar;96(4):434–45.

53 Mazerolle SM, Scruggs IC, Casa DJ, Burton LJ, McDermott BP, Armstrong LE, et al. Current knowledge, attitudes, and practices of certified athletic trainers regarding recognition and treatment of exertional heat stroke. *J Athl Train* 2010 Mar;45(2):170–80.

54 DeMartini JK, Casa DJ, Stearns R, Belval L, Crago A, Davis R, et al. Effectiveness of cold water immersion in the treatment of exertional heat stroke at the Falmouth road race. *Med Sci Sports Exerc* 2015 Feb;47(2):240–5.

INDEX

Note: Page numbers in *italics* and **bold** refer to figures and tables respectively.

acclimation *see* heat acclimation (HA)
acclimatisation *see* heat acclimatisation
active hyperthermia 89–90
active *vs.* passive HA 109
adaptation threshold 102, 104, *104*, 118
after-drop 131, 138
ageing, thermoregulation and 7, 17–19, *18*, 22
air velocity/flow 33–4, 36, 39, 68, 87
aldosterone 16, 159, 167–8, **168**
alpha waves 82, 91, 93–4
ambient temperatures, effect of high 64–78; on cognitive function 86–90; on intermittent exercise 67–8; on neuromuscular performance 71–2; on prolonged exercise performance 68–71, *69*, *71*, 72–6; on sprint exercise performance 66, *67*, 67–8
anticipatory thermoregulation 73–4
arginine vasopressin 159, 162, 166, 167–8, **168**, 171, 173, 175
arousal: alpha waves linked with 82; beta waves linked with 83; cognitive function linked with 89, 91, 94; defined 82; dopamine linked with 74
asymptomatic hyponatremia 173–4
attention, in cognitive function 83, 85, 88–9, 91, 93, 96
aural/tympanic temperature 44–5; *vs.* brain temperature 45

autonomic thermoregulation 6, 9–10, 19
axillary temperature 45

behavioural thermoregulation 6, 9–10, 19–20, *20*, 21
beta waves 83, 91, 93
body mass change **163**, **164**, 166
body temperature measurement considerations 40
brain: structure of *92*; temperature 41, 45

capacity test 64, 70, 74, 110, 143, 169
cardiac output 12–14, *13*
cardiovascular drift 13–14, *14*, 167
cardiovascular responses to exercise performed in hot environment 12–15; cardiac output 12–14, *13*; cardiovascular drift 13–14, *14*; cerebral blood flow 15; heart rate 12–14, *13*; muscle blood flow 14–15; skin blood flow 12; splanchnic blood flow 15; stroke volume 12–14, *13*
cardiovascular stability, effect of heat acclimation on 113
Celsius (°C) 34
central fatigue theory 65, 74–5, *75*
central governor theory 65, 73–4
central sulcus *92*
cerebellum *92*
cerebral blood flow 15
cerebral cortex *92*
Clo 7, 21

closed-loop tests 65, 70
clothing: head and neck garments for cooling 141–2; heat acclimation by wearing more layers 109–10; ice vests for cooling 138–41, *139, 140*; thermoregulation and 7, 21–2, 23
cognitive function: areas of 84–5; attention in 83, 85, 88–9, 91, 93, 96; defined 83, 84–5; effect of hot ambient conditions on 86–90; effect of hyperthermia on 90–5; effect of hypohydration on 172–3; effect of pre-cooling on 146–7; executive function in 83, 84, 88–9, 95; human brain and 91–2; impaired by severe increases in core body temperature 91–4; improved by moderate increases in core body temperature 91; maximal adaptability model *93*; memory in 83–5, *86*, 88–90, 92, 94; minimising effect of exercise in heat 84, 95; other effects of hot ambient conditions on 94–5; psychomotor speed in 83, 85; social and emotional cognition in 83, 85; tests 85–6, *86*
Cohen's *d* 132, 134, 136, 146
cold beverage ingestion **133**, 144–5, **152**
cold-water immersion 137–8; cold beverage ingestion 145; to cool core body temperature 138, 145, 197–200, *199*; cooling before exercise 134; defined 131; forearm/hand 197; mixed-method cooling 145–6; pre-cooling 147, 148; summarising **133, 152, 196**; for treating heat illnesses and injuries **196**, 197–200, *199*; whole-body water immersion 147, 201
computer-based cognitive function tests *86*
conductive heat transfer, in heat balance equation 9
constant work HA 108
controlled hyperthermia 103, 108–9, 123, **126**
convective heat transfer, in heat balance equation 7, 8–9
cooling 131–52; effect of pre-cooling on cognitive performance in heat 146–7; in elite sport 131, 134, *134*; of elite time-trial cyclist 132, 147–9; before exercise 134–6, *135*, 147–8; before and during exercise *135*, 136; during exercise *135*, 136, 148–9; interventions *see* cooling interventions; methods *see* cooling methods; strategies, summarising most commonly used **133, 152**; when to cool 134–6

cooling interventions **196**, 196–200, *197, 199*; cold packs **196**; cold showers 195, 196, **196**; ice sheets 196, **196**; ice towels 136, 141, 143, 146, 196, **196**; passive rest **196**, 198; *see also* cold-water immersion; ice vests
cooling jackets *see* ice vests
cooling methods 137–46; cold beverage ingestion 144–5; cold-water immersion 137–8; fan cooling 142–3, *143*; head and neck garments 141–2; ice vests 138–41, *139, 140*; menthol cooling 143–4; mixed-method cooling 145–6; summarising **133, 152**
cooling vests *see* ice vests
core body temperature: adaptations, decay in 119; after-drop 131, 138; ageing and thermoregulation 17; behavioural thermoregulation 19–20; cardiovascular responses to exercise performed in hot environment 12, 13, *13*, 113; clothing and acclimation 109–10; clothing and thermoregulation 22; cognitive function impaired by severe increases in 91–4; cognitive function improved by moderate increases in 91; cold beverage ingestion 145; cold-water immersion 138, 145, 197–200, *199*; cooling rate, defined 187; critical core temperature 65, 72–4; effect of heat acclimation on 113 *see also* heat acclimation (HA); exertional heatstroke 188, 192–3; fan cooling 142; head and neck cooling garments 141; heat adaptation 111; heat reacclimation 120–1; heat-related injury and illness 189, 192–3, 194, 196–202, *197*; heat storage 7–10; hyperthermia 71, 87, 88–90, 108–9; hypohydration 167–8, 171; hypoxia 117; ice slurry ingestion 145, 148; ice vests 139; intermittent exercise and repeated sprint performance 67–8; isothermic hyperthermia 103; mean time taken to cool *197*, 197–8; measuring *see* core body temperature, measuring; molecular responses to exercise performed in hot environment 17; prescriptive zone 7; responses to exercise performed in hot environment 10–11, *11*; sweat responses 16, 114; temperature and cooler temperatures 116; thermal impulses 103, *104*; wet-bulb globe temperature 36
core body temperature, measuring 40–5; assessment summary **59**; aural/tympanic

temperature 44–5; axillary temperature 45; brain temperature 41, 45; gastrointestinal temperature 43–4; mean body temperature 47–8; oesophageal temperature 42; oral temperature 44; physiological strain index 48–50, **49**; pulmonary arterial temperature 41–2; rectal temperature 43; reference table summarising 57, **58**; sites commonly used for *41, 42*; skin temperature 45–7, *46*; thermal comfort 50–1, **52**; thermal sensation 50; thermal sensation scales 50, **51**
corpus callosum *92*
critical core temperature 65, 72–4
cross-adaptation 115–18; hypoxia 117–18; temperate and cooler conditions 116–17
cross-tolerance *see* cross-adaptation

DB *see* dry bulb (DB)
dehydration: defined 159; rehydration 161; *see also* hydration
"do not start" considerations 37–9, *38*
dopamine 74–5, 91, 95, 96
dry bulb (DB) 36
duration of HA 106

EAH *see* exercise-associated hyponatremia (EAH)
eccrine sweat glands 7, 16
EEG *see* electroencephalography (EEG)
effect sizes: Cohen's *d* 132, 134, 136, 146; defined 132; in forest plot *112*; Hedges' *g* 132, *135*, 136; of pre- and per-cooling approaches 134–6, *135*; for sweat rate 114
electroencephalography (EEG) 83, 90, 93–4
elite athlete, optimising heat acclimation for 103, 122
elite sport, cooling in 131, 134, *134*
elite time-trial cyclist: per-cooling 148–9; pre-cooling 147–8
emotional bias 85
emotion recognition 85
endotoxemia 15, 187–8, 189, 192, 193, 194–5
euhydration: defined 160; osmolality 165; post-exercise 175; pre-exercise 174; trials 171; urine colour 166, 177; urine specific gravity 165
evaporative heat transfer, in heat balance equation 7, 8
executive function, in cognitive function 83, 84, 88–90, 95

exercise-associated hyponatremia (EAH) 173–4
exercise-associated muscle cramps 188, 189, 191, **205**
exercise performance, effect of high ambient temperatures on prolonged 68–71, *69, 71*, 72–6; anticipatory thermoregulation 73–4; central fatigue theory 74–5, *75*; central governor theory 74; critical core temperature hypothesis 72–3, 74; decay in performance improvements 120; heat acclimation 110–11; hypohydration **168**, 168–72; integrative model 75–6; sprinting 66, *67*, 67–8
exertional heat exhaustion 188, 189, 191–2, 200–1, **205**
exertional heatstroke 188, 189, 192–3, 194, 200–1, **205**
external cooling 132, 137, 141

Fahrenheit (°F) 34
fan cooling **133**, 142–3, *143*, **152**
fine motor skill *86*
fluid balance, effect of heat acclimation on markers of 114
fluid balance regulation 160–2; dehydration and rehydration 161; thirst 162; total body water 160–1
fMRI *see* functional magnetic resonance imaging (fMRI)
fourth ventricle *92*
frequency of HA 106
frontal lobe 83, 92, *92*, 94
functional magnetic resonance imaging (fMRI) 90, 92

gamma waves 91
gastrointestinal temperature 43–4
globe thermometer (GT) 36
golden half hour 196
gross motor skill *86*
GT *see* globe thermometer (GT)

HA *see* heat acclimation (HA)
head and neck garments **133**, 141–2, **152**
heart rate 12–14, *13*
heat acclimation (HA) 102–26, *104*; on a budget 103, 121; critical core temperature hypothesis 72; decay *see* heat acclimation (HA) decay; defined 102; effect of, on cardiovascular stability 113; effect of, on core body and skin temperature 113; effect of, on exercise

performance 110–11; effect of, on markers of fluid balance 114; effect of, on ratings of perceived exertion and thermal sensation 115; effect of, on sweat responses 114; heat acclimatisation *vs.* 103–5, *104*; heat reacclimation 120–3; hypoxia 117–18; methods *see* heat acclimation (HA) methods; molecular basis to 115; optimising, for elite athlete 103, 122; for performance in other conditions (cross-adaptation) 115–18; physiological and perceptual responses to 111–16; temperature and cooler conditions 116–17; type *see* heat acclimation (HA) phenotype; *see also* heat adaptation

heat acclimation (HA) decay 102, 103, 116, 118–21; in core body temperature adaptations 119; in heart rate adaptations 118–19; in performance improvements 120; in sweat response adaptations 119–20

heat acclimation (HA) methods 105–10, **126**; duration 106; frequency 106; intensity 107; type 107–10

heat acclimation (HA) phenotype 107–10; active *vs.* passive HA 109; constant work HA 108; isothermic/controlled hyperthermia HA 108–9; self-regulated/self-paced work HA 108; wearing more layers 109–10

heat acclimatisation 102–26; defined 102; heat acclimation *vs.* 103–5, *104*; heat stress intensity 107; methods **126**; naturally occurring 115

heat adaptation: classic markers of 111; cross-adaptation 115–18; Forest plot summarising effect of *112*; integrated overview of *112*; osmolality 111, *112*; physiological and perceptual responses to 111–18; *see also* heat acclimation (HA)

heat balance equation $(S = M \pm W - E \pm C \pm K \pm R)$ 7–9; S = storage of body heat 7–9; M = metabolic heat production 8; W = work 8; E = evaporative heat transfer 7, 8; C = convective heat transfer 7, 8–9; K = conductive heat transfer 9; R = radiant heat transfer 9

heat exhaustion, exertional 188, 189, 191–2, 200–1, **205**

heat reacclimation (HR) 103, 120–3

heat-related injury and illness 187–205; cooling interventions **196**, 196–200, *197*, *199*; diagnosing 188, 200–1; endotoxemia 15, 187–8, 189, 192,

193, 194–5; exercise-associated muscle cramps 188, 189, 191, **205**; exertional heat exhaustion 188, 189, 191–2, 200–1, **205**; exertional heatstroke 188, 189, 192–3, 194, 200–1, **205**; golden half hour 196; minimise likelihood of 189, 201–2; preventing 193–5; quick reference table for heat illness **205**; sunburn 188, 189, 190–1, 192, 194, 195, 202, **205**; treating major 195–200; treating minor 195

heat-shock proteins 7, 17, 109, 115, 117

heat storage 7–10; heat balance equation 7–9; regulating 9–10

heatstroke, exertional 188, 189, 192–3, 194, 200–1, **205**

Hedges' *g* 132, *135*, 136

humidity, defined 33

humidity, effect of: on intermittent exercise 67–8; on neuromuscular performance 71–2; on prolonged exercise performance 68–71, *69*, *71*, 72–6; on sprint exercise performance 66, *67*, 67–8

hydration 159–82; dehydration, defined 159; exercise-associated hyponatremia 173–4; fluid balance regulation 160–2; optimising, for team sport athlete 160, 177–8; status *see* hydration status, measuring; strategies *see* hydration strategies; *see also* hypohydration

hydration status, measuring 162–7; body mass change **163**, **164**, 166; clinical variables 167; in field 160, 177; osmolality of plasma and urine 163, **163**, **164**, 165; summary of **163**; urine colour **163**, **164**, 165–6; urine specific gravity **163**, **164**, 165

hydration strategies 174–6; per-exercise 174–5; point-counterpoint discussion 176, **176**; post-exercise 175; pre-exercise 174; prescribed *vs.* "to thirst" 176; quick reference **181**

hyperhydration 159–60, 161, 166

hyperthermia: active 89–90; cognitive function influenced by 90–5; controlled 103, 108–9, 123, **126**; isothermic 103, 107, 108–9, 123, **126**; passive 88–9

hypertonic fluid 160, 165, 174

hypohydration: cold water ingestion **133**; defined 160; effects of, on cognitive performance in heat 172–3; effects of, on exercise performance in heat **168**, 168–72; exertional heat exhaustion 191; exertional muscle cramps 194, **205**;

fluid balance regulation 161; impaired
cognitive function linked to 89;
involuntary 162; osmolality 165;
physiological effects of 167–8, **168**;
summary of **176**; thirst sensation 114,
162, 171–2; trials 171; urine colour 165;
volitional fluid consumption 114
hyponatremia: asymptomatic 173–4;
defined 160; exercise-associated 173–4;
exertional heat cramps 195; main risk
factors for 173; summary of **176**;
symptomatic 173–4; WBGT "do not
start" considerations 38
hypothalamic–pituitary–adrenal axis stress
response 107
hypothalamus 9, 15, 19, 45, *92*, 107, *112*,
162, 167
hypotonic fluid 160, 165, 171, 174, 175
hypovolaemia 161, 162, 165
hypoxia 117–18

ice jackets *see* ice vests
ice vests 138–41, *139*, *140*; Arctic Heat
139, *139*; defined 132; measuring
perceived thermal strain and comfort
52; *vs.* mixed-method cooling 145–6;
per-cooling 136, 148; pre-cooling 136,
147–8; summarising **133**, **152**, **196**;
weight of 139
illness, heat-related *see* heat-related injury
and illness
injury, heat-related *see* heat-related injury
and illness
integrative model 65, 75–6
intensity of HA 107
interhalamic adhesion *92*
intermittent exercise, effect of high
ambient temperatures and humidity on
repeated 67–8
internal cooling 132, 137, 144–5
isothermic/controlled hyperthermia
HA 108–9
isothermic HA 111, 113, 123
isothermic hyperthermia 103, 108–9,
123, **126**
isotonic fluid 160, 165, 171, 174

Kelvin (K) 34

laboratory-based environmental chamber
102, 103
lipopolysaccharide (LPS) 188, 193, 194
liquid-cooled cooling jacket *140*
long-term heat acclimation (LTHA) 103,
106, 110–11, *112*, 114, 122

marathon: heat and 34–5, *35*, 53–4, *53–4*;
optimal environmental conditions for
world record attempt 66, 76
maximal adaptability model *93*
mean body temperature 47–8
mean skin temperature *46*, 46–7
medula *92*
memory, in cognitive function 83–5, *86*,
88–90, 92, 94; defined 85; episodic
memory 85; recognition memory 85;
working memory 83–5, *86*, 88–90,
92, 94
mental flexibility, in executive function 84
menthol cooling **133**, 143–4, **152**
metabolic heat production, in heat balance
equation 8
mid-cooling *see* per-cooling
mixed-method cooling 145–6
moderate-term heat acclimation (MTHA)
103, 106, 110–11, *112*, 113, 114, 124
molecular basis to heat acclimation
115, 118
molecular responses to heat 17
MTHA *see* moderate-term heat acclimation
(MTHA)
muscle blood flow 14–15
muscle cramps, exercise-associated 188, 189,
191, **205**

neuromuscular performance, effect of
high ambient temperatures and humidity
on 71–2
neurotransmitters 65, 74, 91
noradrenaline 65, 74–5

occipital lobe 83, 92, *92*
oesophageal temperature 42
oral temperature 44
osmolality: defined 160; dehydration 161;
in euhydration 160; in heat adaptation
111, *112*; hydration status, measurement
of **163**; of hypertonic fluid 160; in
hypohydration 160; hypohydration and
167–8, 170, 172; of hypotonic fluid
160; of isotonic fluid 160; post-exercise
hydration strategies 175; prescribed *vs.*
"to thirst" 177; thirst sensation 162;
urine and 163–6, **164**, 177

paired associates learning test 85, *86*
parietal lobe 83, 92, *92*
parieto-occipital sulcus *92*
passive HA, active *vs.* 109
passive hyperthermia 88–9
passive rest **196**, 198

perception-based heat strain index 52
per-cooling: cold beverage ingestion 145;
cold-water immersion 137; defined
132; effect sizes of 134–6, *135*; elite
time-trial cyclist 148–9; head and neck
cooling garments 141, 142; ice vests
140, 141; mixed-method cooling 136;
summary of **133**
per-exercise (hydration strategy) 174–5, **181**
performance tests 64, 65, 70, 73, 74,
110, 171
physiological adaptation *104*, 109, 116,
121–3, 202
physiological strain index 48–50, **49**
pineal gland *92*
pituitary gland *92*, *112*, 167
pons *92*
post-exercise (hydration strategy) 175, **181**
pre-cooling 134–6, 146–7; cold-water
immersion 137; defined 132; effect
sizes of 134–6, *135*; effects of, on
cognitive performance in heat 146–7;
elite time-trial cyclist 147–8; head and
neck cooling garments 141; ice vests
140, 141; mixed-method cooling 136;
summary of **133**
predicted heat strain model 39
pre-exercise (hydration strategy) 174, **181**
prescriptive zone 7, 11, 70
preseason training and heat 35, 55
problem-based learning 1
prolonged exercise performance, effect of
high ambient temperatures and humidity
on 68–71, *69*, *71*, 72–6; anticipatory
thermoregulation 73–4; central fatigue
theory 74–5, *75*; central governor theory
74; critical core temperature hypothesis
72–3, 74; integrative model 75–6
psychomotor speed, in cognitive function
83, 85
pulmonary arterial temperature 41–2

radiant heat 34, 36, 76
radiant heat transfer, in heat balance
equation 7, 9
rapid visual information processing *86*, 146
ratings of perceived exertion (RPE)
19–20, *20*, 91, 107, 115, 136,
142, 144, 170–1
reaction time: hyperthermia 88, 90, 95;
hypohydration 172; pre-cooling 146; test
85, *86*, 95
reciprocal inhibition model 10
rectal temperature 43
refractometer 160, 165, 177

rehydration 161; defined 160; heat illnesses
and injuries 195, 201; hypohydration
170; post-exercise 175
response inhibition, in executive
function 84
reticular activating system *92*
reuptake inhibitor 65, 74–5
RPE *see* ratings of perceived
exertion (RPE)

self-regulated/self-paced work HA 108
short-term heat acclimation (STHA) 103,
106, 107, 110–11, *112*, 113, 114, 124
skin blood flow 12
skin temperature measurement 45–7, *46*
social and emotional cognition, in cognitive
function 83, 85
spatial working memory *86*
spinal cord 9, *92*
splanchnic blood flow 15
sprint exercise performance, effect of high
ambient temperatures 66–8, *67*
STHA *see* short-term heat acclimation
(STHA)
storage of body heat, in heat balance
equation 7–9
stroke volume 12–14, *13*
Stroop test *85*
sudomotor capacity 114
sudomotor response to heat 16, 114,
145, 149
sudomotor threshold 114
sunburn 188, 189, 190–1, 192, 194,
195, 202
sustained attention 85
sweat loss and rate 114, **182**
sweat responses: adaptations, heat
acclimation decay in 119–20; core body
temperature 16, 114; exercise performed
in hot environment 15–16
symptomatic hyponatremia 173–4

thalamus *92*
thermal comfort, measuring 50–1, **52**
thermal impulse 103, *104*, 106, 108, 111,
113, 118, 123, 202
thermal sensation 50, **51**; measuring 50;
scales **51**, 52
thermal strain: defined 34; estimating from
thermal stress data 39–40; marathon and
heat 34–5, *35*, 53–4, *53–4*; measuring
see thermal strain, measuring; preseason
training and heat 35, 55
thermal strain, measuring 40–50;
body temperature measurement

considerations 40; mean body temperature 47–8; perceived thermal strain and comfort 50–2; perception-based heat strain index 52; physiological strain index 48–50, **49**; sites commonly used for *41*, *42*; skin temperature measurement 45–7, *46*; thermal comfort 50–1, **52**; thermal sensation 50, **51**; *see also* core body temperature, measuring

thermal stress: data, estimating thermal strain from 39–40; defined 34; marathon and heat 34–5, *35*, 53–4, *53–4*; measuring *see* thermal stress, measuring; predicted heat strain model 39; preseason training and heat 35, 55; universal thermal climate index 39–40

thermal stress, measuring 36–9; parameters 36; predicted heat strain model 39; summary of 40; universal thermal climate index 39–40; wet-bulb globe temperature 36–9

thermoreceptors 9, 19, 50, *112*, 145

thermoregulation 6–26; ageing 7, 17–19, *18*, 22; anticipatory 73–4; behavioural 19–20, *20*; autonomic 6, 9–10, 19; cardiovascular responses to exercise performed in hot environment 12–15; clothing 7, 21–2, 23; core body temperature responses to exercise performed in hot environment 10–11, *11*; heat storage 7–10; molecular responses to exercise performed in hot environment 17; sweat responses to exercise performed in hot environment 15–16

theta waves 84, 91, 93–4

thirst 114, 162, 167, 171–2

threshold: adaptation 102, 104, *104*, 118; sudomotor 114

total body water 160–1

ultraviolet radiation (UVA and UVB) 188, 190, 194, 202

universal thermal climate index 39–40

urine: colour **163**, **164**, 165–6; osmolality of 163, **163**, **164**, 165

urine specific gravity (USG) **163**, **164**, 165

UVA and UVB (ultraviolet radiation) 188, 190, 194, 202

visuomotor accuracy *86*, 89, 172

voluntary activation 65, 71–2, 74

wet bulb (WB) 36

wet-bulb globe temperature (WBGT) 36–40; defined 34, 37; "do not start" considerations 37–9, *38*; equations 37; issues with 37; thermometers 36

whole-body water immersion 147, 201

wind chill 9

work, in heat balance equation 8

working memory, in executive function 83–5, *86*, 88–90, 92, 94

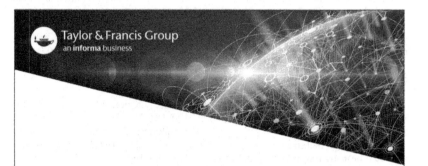